The Blues (Splanchnic Neurasthenia)
Causes and Cure

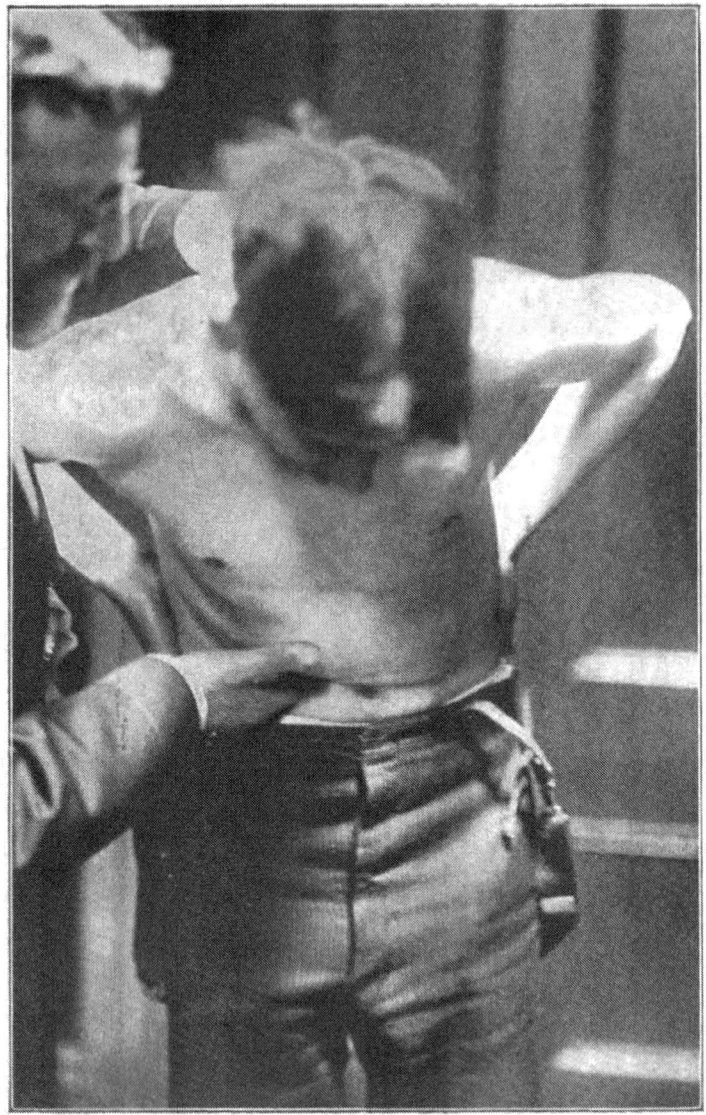

Fig. 16.—The author's method of palpating the liver.   See page 192.

THE BLUES

(SPLANCHNIC NEURASTHENIA)

CAUSES AND CURE

BY

ALBERT ABRAMS, A.M., M.D. (Heidelberg), F.R.M.S.

CONSULTING PHYSICIAN, DENVER NATIONAL HOSPITAL FOR CONSUMP-
TIVES, THE MOUNT ZION AND THE FRENCH HOSPITALS, SAN FRAN-
CISCO; PRESIDENT OF THE EMANUEL SISTERHOOD POLYCLINIC;
FORMERLY PROFESSOR OF PATHOLOGY AND DIRECTOR OF
THE MEDICAL CLINIC, COOPER MEDICAL COLLEGE,
SAN FRANCISCO

ILLUSTRATED

NEW YORK.

E. B. TREAT AND COMPANY

241–243 WEST 23D STREET

1904

PREFACE.

THE object of this volume is to direct reference to a new and heretofore undescribed variety of nerve exhaustion, which I have designated as, *Splanchnic Neurasthenia.* This special form of nerve weakness is characterized by paroxysms of depression of varying duration, and which are specified popularly as "*the blues.*" The recognition of this special form of neurasthenia is of more than theoretic interest. One cannot say of it as did the mathematician, who, having demonstrated a new mathematical theory, thanked God that it could not be of the slightest utility to any living soul. A mere theory may be of interest to members of our profession, but the layman asks science for results. The recognition of splanchnic neurasthenia and the factors involved in its causation, imply our ability to cope with the evil and offer to the sufferers not only amelioration, but cure in many instances. My experience with neurasthenics has extended over a period of many years, and I know of no variety of neurasthenia which is more amenable to treatment than the splanchnic form. Various writers have hinted at an abdominal form of neurasthenia, but to my knowledge they have ignored the true source of origin. A perusal of the subject matter of this volume will show that I have referred the origin of splanchnic neu-

3

rasthenia, in brief, to a congestion of the intra-abdominal veins. Man is distinguished from all other mammals by his erect posture. "If an intelligent extramundane" says Campbell, "were to see man for the first time in the horizontal posture, it would never occur to him that it is natural for him to be erect. There is something incongruous in an animal built on the longitudinal plan standing and progressing upon one end of its long axis." The erect posture of man places him at a disadvantage in several directions, notably, however, by increasing the height of the blood column with a corresponding increase of gravity on the circulation, thus causing the blood to gravitate into the intra-abdominal veins. Among the many resources of Nature to combat this tendency, the vigor of the abdominal muscles is paramount. The tonicity of the muscles in question is impaired by mal-hygienic clothing, occupation, disease, lack of exercise and a host of other conditions. Even a physiologic condition like pregnancy conduces to relaxation of the abdominal wall and pendulous belly, the so-called *hänge-bauch* of the Germans, and yet no one dreams of restoring the defective musculature after pregnancy by well directed exercises. The sports of the ancient Greeks were specially directed toward development of the abdominal muscles. In the sculptural works of the old masters, the abdominal muscles are reproduced with as much accuracy as the other muscles of the body, and it is reasonable to assume, contrasting the art of the ancients with that of the modern sculptors, that the decadence of the abdominal muscles is a modern heritage; and so are hemorrhoids, constipation, hernia, and a multitude of other evils that may be traced to enfeebled abdominal muscles. It is surprising how little can be achieved by feeble abdominal muscles, and how much when the latter are developed by exercises. Individuals who would flinch when the slightest abdominal pressure was made, could after a few months' use of the abdominal exerciser, throw heavy individuals seated on their abdomens, up and down, as serenely as though they were rubber balls. This exerciser permits essentially of tractions being made by the abdomen, although the exercises may be made in different directions. The abdominal exerciser is likewise available in developing other muscles of the body. In this connection, the experiments of Prof. W. G. Anderson, of Yale University, may be recalled with profit. The latter succeeded in practically weighing the result of a thought's action. A student was placed on a "muscle-bed," poised on a balance so that the center of gravity of his body was exactly over its center. When the student was directed to solve mathematical problems, the increased weight of blood at his head changed his center of gravitation and caused an immediate dip of the balance to that side. The student was further directed to imagine himself going through leg gymnastics. As the feats were mentally performed, one by one, the blood flamed to the limbs in sufficient quantities to tip the balance, according to the movement thought of. His experiments warrant the conclusion, that the important thing in all exercises is the mental effort put forth: thus, walking is inadequate exercise for brain workers, as it is so purely automatic that it does not call the blood from congested brain centers, which continue solving intellectual problems. A run, a brisk walk, with a definite object necessitating the thought of speed, will send the blood to the legs and build them up. There are a large number of gastric and intestinal affections with bizarre and protean symptoms, designated respectively as gastric and intestinal neuroses, but which in reality owe their genesis to a congestion of the intra-abdominal veins. Such affections are essentially forms of splanchnic neurasthenia and are specially amenable to the treatment suggested in this book. The affections in question often produce only local symptoms confined to the abdominal sympathetic, and may never extend beyond the abdominal region to implicate the central nervous system. The treatment I have advocated for the cure of splanchnic neurasthenia is based on purely physiological reasoning. My exposition of the subject of general neurasthenia I have purposely treated cursorily, as it was my intention to employ it as a medium only in introducing my special subject—splanchnic neurasthenia.

ALBERT ABRAMS.

S. W. COR. VAN NESS AVE. AND CALIFORNIA ST.,
SAN FRANCISCO, CAL., JAN., 1904.

CONTENTS.

CHAPTER I.

THE BLUES.

CHAPTER II.

GENERAL IRRITANTS OF NEURASTHENIA.

CHAPTER III.

SPECIAL IRRITANTS OF NEURASTHENIA.

CHAPTER IV.

THE GENERAL AND SPECIAL SYMPTOMS OF NEURASTHENIA.

CHAPTER V.

CHAPTER VI.

CHAPTER VII.

CHAPTER VIII.

APPENDIX.

LIST OF ILLUSTRATIONS.

11

THE BLUES.

CHAPTER I.

THE BLUES.

THE BLUES, AND ITS ALLIED CONDITION NEURASTHENIA.— HEREDITY AS A FACTOR IN THE NERVOUS CONSTITUTION.— PERSONAL EFFORT AS AN ELEMENT IN RESISTING AND OVER- COMING AN UNSTABLE NERVOUS SYSTEM.

RUSKIN, in his "Thoughts of Beauty," is sponsor for the epigram, "God has employed color in His creation as the unvarying accompaniment of all that is purest, most innocent and most precious." Ruskin, evidently never had a "fit" of the blues. Why blue has been the color parodied to illustrate despondency is beyond my ken, for blue has been apostrophized by the painter, poet and litterateur as something expres- sive of heaven, the firmament, truth, constancy, and fidelity. The medical lexicographer pays no tribute to the blues, notwithstanding the fact, that it is se- curely incorporated in the vocabulary of every-day life. I am with aforethought constrained to employ the term "blues" as it appeals with cogent signifi- cance to the sufferer, and for the additional reason that medical art has not truly interpreted its real pathology nor substituted for it, in its nosology, a better or more technical name. The individual with the blues is

13

never an object of compassion. This luxury is denied him. Those nearest and dearest to him make him the butt of their ridicule and ascribe his varied and obscure symptoms to an undue indulgence of the imagination. Driven to despair, he seeks a physician, and the latter may or may not examine him; he may graciously deign to feel his pulse and examine his tongue, and then dismiss him with a prescription for a nerve tonic, and the erudite admonition, "not to become a crank." Physicians are often astute philosophers in sickness, but such philosophy usually concerns the sickness of the other fellow. Sydenham, who loved his profession so well, was wont to observe that, "the medical art could not be learned so well and so surely as by use and experience; and that he who would pay the nicest and most accurate attention to the symptoms of distempers would succeed best in finding out the true means of cure." And Plato contended that medicine was an art which considered the constitution of the patient and had principles of action and reason in each case. There is no symptom which has not a cause for its existence, and though the imagination prove operative in exaggerating its significance, this merely proves that it is in itself not in a state of health. "No one," avers Lavénge, "can be a hypochondriac at pleasure." The unfortunate sufferer of the blues is acutely susceptible to any imputation which discredits the honesty of his statements, and, apprehending no relief from his symptoms, soon falls into the "slough of despond." Such persons never feel "just right"; their sleep is disturbed and the morning heralds the periodical depression and the unconsoling thought of unfitness for the routine work of the day. Memory becomes defective and loss of reason is apprehended. Then follow sexual disturbances, indigestion, constipation, vague head sensations, palpitation of the heart, phobias and a train of obscure and indefinite symptoms which baffle interpretation and add immeasurably to the suffering of the individual. The picture of the neurasthenic presents an insane revelry of the organs with the mind in the background, perceiving physiologic as pathologic functions. In the foreground stands the physician, a solemn witness of the scene, and whose face, the theatre of his soul, betrays the thought; how little power his art has given him to interpret objectively what is so acutely cognizant to the unfortunate sufferer. The stomach of the patient may cause him untold agony, yet analyze his stomach contents and you will find that there is no anomaly of digestion; examine his palpitating heart which, with every thump, increases his anxiety, and you listen to tones modified neither in intensity nor in cadence; and thus you proceed to examine organ after organ and there is nothing revealed; your examination is negative and your negative examination sustains your diagnosis; you may call it what you will, neurasthenia or the blues. An attack of the blues is nought else but an acute neurasthenia or an aperiodic exacerbation of chronic neurasthenia. Neurasthenia having been firmly established in medical technology, it will be under this name that the subject will be further discussed.

Dr. Beard, of New York, is the godfather of neurasthenia, having Hellenized its correlative nerve weakness. A medley of terms have been suggested to specify the varied symptoms and accompaniments of reduced nerve force, viz: hypochondriasis, nervousness, brain strain, nervous waste, nervous prostration,

nervous exhaustion, nervous breakdown, spinal irritation, etc., etc.   The foregoing terms impose on us the
assumption that we are here dealing with an essentially
nervous disease, but further consideration of the subject
may convince us, as we proceed, that in many examples
of the affection, and I may add the great majority, the
nervous symptoms are merely secondary.   The cause
may be resident elsewhere in the organism, the nervous
system as the point of least resistance, merely reacting
to repeated stimuli, like the rock which is pierced by
the drop of water; not by its force, but by its frequency.
The preceding view assumes, then, that two essential
factors are necessary in the genesis of neurasthenia,
viz: an *enfeebled nervous system* and an incentive, *the
irritant.*

The tale of every neurasthenic may be written in
four chapters: 1. The sins of the fathers.   2. The
birth of a neurotic.   3. Struggle for existence on deficient nerve capital.   4. A bankrupt nervous system.
Throughout the narrative, the continuity of human
folly remains unsevered.   " Our lives," says Darwin,
" are but a bundle of consequences; our present is but
the outcome of the past."

The patient who solicits the counsel of the physician
submits himself as a problemn for analysis; his contemporaneous symptoms proving only a link in the
genetic chain.   The physician, like the ontogenist and
phylogenist respectively concerns himself not only with
the evolution of the individual, but with his ancestral
development.   The question of heredity* as a factor in
neurasthenia is an important one.   Many modern
neurologists contend that heredity is responsible for
the majority of neurasthenics, and one prominent writer

* Appendix, note 12.

recently demonstrated that in one hundred consecutive cases of neurasthenia, a neurotic history could be elicited in 70 per cent. of the cases. I feel confident in asserting that if one hundred consecutive patients came to me for the relief of so plebeian an ailment as corns, I would likewise find no difficulty in obtaining a history of morbid inheritance in a still larger percentage of cases. We comprehend, by neurotic heredity, a number of nervous diseases of direct hereditary character, transmitted from generation to generation. The hereditary taint may vary in degree from epilepsy and insanity to the less serious heritage, neurasthenia. The indications of a neurotic heredity, known as stigmata, may be manifested by defects of moral sense, of memory, attention, will, or judgment. The stigmata of the degenerate may be physical, psychic or both. All writers who have made a psycho-anthropologic study of degenerates do not attach the same significance to physical stigmata as does Lombroso. The chief physical stigmata are: cranial and facial deviation, recession of the lower jaw, large or small mouth and thick lips, abnormally shaped and misplaced ears, defective and misplaced teeth, and high palate.

Criminal anthropologists find such deformities very common, although there are criminals who show no peculiarities, a type referred to by Lombroso, as, "the criminal man." Unless the physical stigma has attained such a degree of structural anomaly as to impair the normal function of a part, no great importance is attached to it. Some of the psychic stigmata are the following: 1. Precocity or retarded evolution of intellect. 2. Extreme changeableness and irritability. 3. Exaggerated consciousness and a fanatical religious zeal or great moral depravity. 4. Intense egotism

2

with no regard for the feeling of others.   5. Extravagant and cranky motives and desires.   6. One-sided talents and disproportionate development of mental faculties.   It was Hawthorne, I believe, who said, "Once in every half century, at longest, a family should . . . forget all about its ancestors."

The hereditarian contends that "the gods visit the sins of the fathers upon the children": "That we are omnibuses in which all our ancestors ride;" and, "that the life of each individual is, in some real sense, a continuation of the lives of his ancestors." The pessimistic fatalism expressed in the preceding epigrams seeks to eliminate the personal equation as a factor in disease, thus limiting the responsibility to heredity. We must not forget, however, that the autocratic reasoning of the hereditarian is by no means final, nor must we blindly submit to a ruling which would deprive the unfortunate neurotic of all hope.

A recent writer, Prof. Putnam,[1] attempts to explode the baneful argument of the hereditarian, and assures us that a just regard for the laws of hygiene will help to avert disease. He says that "fortunately for the educational outlook, the evidence has begun to accumulate that a morbid inheritance is not the inevitably crushing and baneful thing that it has been thought. We come into the world, each one a being of limited capacity, but, in other respects, free to become what circumstances make us, and responsible, to the extent of our capacity, for our lot. We bring no ticket-of-leave which stamps us as drunkards or maniacs on probation, but we do bear, in the histories of our ancestors, a certificate that hints by what efforts and by what avoidances we can make ourselves reasonable successes in our respective lines. There is no original sin, and not even, as it seems to me, original propensity, but only original capacity and original limitation, and even limitation is only another name for latent capacity."

Let us select consumption as a paradigm of an hereditary disease, and learn to what degree personal effort is responsible in averting it. The modern physician assumes correctly that there is an inherited predisposition to pulmonary tuberculosis, and that the susceptible individual, unlike the neurasthenic, betrays unmistakable objective stigmata of such predisposition. If the physician, however, were dominated by the pessimistic fatalism of the hereditarian, he could extend no hope to the individual predisposed to consumption; but fortunately he has weaned himself from the irrational dogmas associated with this dire disease, and he can confidently say to the individual in question, " Lead a regular and hygienic life and you have nothing to fear from the taint of heredity."

To prevent an unstable and mental nervous organization, we must begin with the parents, and exercise always, from birth on, eternal vigilance, which is the only true passport to longevity and freedom from disease. It was Voltaire who said, " If as much care were taken to perpetuate a race of fine men as is done to prevent the mixture of ignoble blood in horses and dogs, the genealogy of every one would be written on his face and displayed in his manners." Homiculture or the physical culture of man corresponds to the means adopted in improving the breed of the lower animals.

In these days, when sentiment and not reason dictates mating, it would prove fatuous to enlist the cooperation of the individual, and there is urgent need for legislative measures in this direction. Sanitary marriages need not detract from the sentiment which is associated with matrimony; on the contrary, they would confer on the matrimonial candidates a boon unattainable by any other means, and the progeny of such marriages would receive health as a heritage, the most sublime gift which parents can bequeath to their children.

Christian civilization need not emulate nor revive the laws of the 'Spartans, but from the latter many valuable lessons could be learned. The Spartans idolized what was beautiful and useful and sought by vigorous means to attain them. The sick were not allowed to marry, but the healthy were compelled to enter wedlock. Bachelors were publicly denounced after a certain age and banished from society. Marriage was not permitted in either sex until the age of maturity. The result of this Spartan system of marriage was to produce for five hundred years the strongest and bravest men and the most beautiful and healthy women that this world has ever known.

The nervous and mental hygiene of the individual begins at birth and ends only with the extinction of life. It consists in the main of making the mind and body insusceptible to environment by imposing conditions which mean bodily discomfort and mental hardship. We must put ourselves in Nature's place and work as Nature works, or, as Hufeland, puts it, "The nearer and truer we are to Mother Earth, and the closer our intercourse with Nature, the closer we approach the source of Eternal youth and health; hence, it it only necessary to understand how nature intended that we should live in order to live long and comfortably; art can do nothing to assist."

SUMMARY.

1. The "blues" is a popular term emp oyed to express a multitude of ill-defined symptoms, mainly nervous, which have not, as yet, been included in the category of diseases.

2. An attack of the blues is an attack of acute neurasthenia or an aperiodic aggravation of chronic nervousness.

3. Nervousness, while expressive of an enfeebled nervous system, is an expression evoked by some irritant resident somewhere in the organism, other than in the nervous apparatus.

4. Heredity may be responsible for the susceptible nervous system, and it devolves on the individual to obey the laws of hygiene and to avail himself "of momentary advantages, however minute, to withstand the effects of conditions which either weaken or improve the status of his vitality."

5. Heredity and environment may be effectually fought by personal effort.

CHAPTER II.

GENERAL IRRITANTS OF NEURASTHENIA.

HOW IRRITANTS OPERATE.—OVERWORK, WORRY, THE ABUSE OF ALCOHOL, BODILY DISEASES &C, AS CAUSES OF NEURASTHENIA.—THE PATHOLOGY OF NEURASTHENIA.—BRAIN CHANGES IN NEURASTHENIA.—FATIGUE NEURASTHENIA.

In the previous chapter, incidental mention was made of the causes of neurasthenia which, having their inception at birth, continue through life and are only extinguished by death. "As the twig is bent, the tree's inclined." The mental and moral education of the child should be our primary concern. It is customary to regard neurasthenia as a disease of adult life, a contention which is as absurd as saying that adults only have a nervous system. The neurasthenic never seems to be rested; that "tired feeling" is always with him, and this susceptibility to fatigue constitutes the primary and fundamental symptom of the disease, and without it the disease cannot be said to exist. It is true that fatigue symptoms soon graduate into sensations of pains and aches, to recur again and again, until they are established as a permanent condition, dominated by a morbid mentality. In childhood, neurasthenia may be expressed wholly by the feeling of tire, and it is only rarely that the morbid physical sensations obtrude themselves sufficiently in consciousness to make the mind a factor in the vicious circle. It has been customary recently to identify nerve force with electricity and if the analogy is not scientifically correct, it will at least subserve our purpose in enabling us to so manipulate our subject matter as to deal with something more tangible than nerve force. A recent writer, O'Brien,[2] says, "I picture the nervous system and its mechanisms in living action before my mind; I see beside it the central telegraph system of New York or London, with its radii of lines and cables, telephonic and telegraphic; its multiple switches, batteries, relays, transformers, condensers, resistances, shunts, duplex and automatic circuits: all this mechanism, like the nervous system, transmitting force and translating intelligence from point to point by terminal instruments which move, talk, write, print, light, inhibit, accelerate and regulate and in one hundred ways doing what is done in the nervous system, and always by means of the same force, the only form of force capable of such vast and varied service."

The voluntary, automatic and reflex movements of a child or adult, the employment of the senses and every thought means the expenditure of so much nerve force. When a muscle is fatigued by voluntary contraction, it involves not only the muscle but the nervous system, and the latter to a larger degree than the former. It is erroneous to suppose that a healthy nervous system can be acquired by vigorous muscular exercise. The latter always means an expenditure of nerve force which may or may not be beyond the capacity of the individual. Many nervous wrecks are recruited from this fallacious argument. Muscular exercise is healthful to the extent of provoking pleasant recreation and relief from mental work. Muscular exercise makes a predatory raid on nerve force which, being thus consumed, limits the mental powers of the individual. The nervous hygiene of childhood embraces the elimination of so many irritants that to enumerate them would be beyond the scope of this work. Suffice it to say, at this time, that tire in the child as well as the adult is the signal of warning. Tire is Nature's call for rest. Heed Nature and there is no danger from any amount of work that we are desirous of doing. The other chief irritants of neurasthenia are: mental overwork associated with anxiety, worry or excitement, the abuse of alcohol, tobacco, coffee, tea, bodily disorders, physiologic factors and moral causes.

MENTAL OVERWORK.—Ruskin, has correctly observed, that, " no great intellectual thing was ever done by great effort; a great thing can only be done by a great man, and he does it without effort. The body's work and the head's work are to be done quietly and comparatively without effort. Neither limbs nor brain are ever to be strained to their utmost. That is not the way in which the greatest quantity of work is to be gotten out of them. They are never to be worked furiously, but with tranquillity and constancy. We are to follow the plough from sunrise to sunset, but not to pull in race boats at the twilight; we shall get no fruit out of that kind of work." The Solomonic rule is not a bad one to follow, viz: eight hours for labor and occupation, eight hours for rest, refreshment and recreation and surcease of all labor, and eight hours for sleep. The nervous system must be made equal to its task. Nerve health depends on a moderate amount of work well diluted with healthful and cheerful recreation. Gibson,[8] expressed a Utopian idea, when he said, " Man is advancing to a stage when he shall no longer

remain a stranger to his own life processes." It would
be better for man were he conscious of his life processes
in the sense of knowing his capacity for work and the
need of rest when that is necessary. Such mental training could be designated as physiologic introspection, and
is the key-note of health. Holmes, in "Over the Tea-
cups" speaks as follows of the curve of health: "It is
a mistake to suppose that the normal state of health is
represented by a straight horizontal line. Independ-
ently of the well-known causes which raise or depress
the standard of vitality, there seems to be—I think I
may venture to say there is—a rhythmic undulation in
the flow of the vital force. The dynamo which furnishes the working powers of consciousness and action
has its annual, its monthly, its diurnal, even its momentary ripples, in the current it furnishes. There
are greater and lesser curves in the movement of every-
day life—a series of ascending and descending movements, a periodicity depending upon the very nature
of the force at work in the living organism. Thus we
have our good seasons and our bad seasons, our good
days and our bad days, life climbing and descending in
long or short undulations, which I have called *the curve
of health.*"

The brain worker who works with discretion knows
that the brain is capable of the greatest amount of
work without fatigue during the early morning hours,
for sleep has served to recuperate a fagged brain.
The discretionate brain worker also knows that there
is a daily ebb and flow of his nerve vigor. From the
early morning hours the ebb of nerve force begins, attaining its maximum discharge in the middle of the
afternoon, a time when the nervously exhausted are
the most weak. The evening meal temporarily stimu-

lates the brain functions, masking as it were the depressed state of the nervous system. Then follows sleep. The brain worker requires more sleep than the laborer. There are certain individuals whose occupations predispose them to neurasthenia. Thus it is, that merchants, professional men, teachers and others furnish large numbers of neurasthenics; their mental application is so profound and intense, that they exceed the limits of human endurance without a conscious knowledge of the fact. Then again, the brain worker is usually a neurasthenic, for, in this strenuous life of ours, mental achievement is only possible with a highly irritable nervous system. " The power of originality in new lines of thought" as Maudsley puts it, "and stepping aside from the beaten track of reflection, is, of itself, a common indication of the insane neurosis."

There are individuals who are incapable of appreciating the great amount of work they really do; they blunt their sense of tire by artificial stimulants and excitement. The latter class of individuals soon become drug habitués or end their lives in asylums as paretics. The predisposing cause of paresis so sententiously expressed by Mickle applies with equal cogency to neurasthenia: " A life absorbed in ambitious projects with all its strongest mental efforts, its long sustained anxieties, deferred hopes, and straining expectation." The individual who seeks to avoid neurasthenia by mental inactivity should hearken to the couplet of Cowper:

" Absence of occupation is not rest,
A mind quite vacant is a mind distressed."

The perpetuation of any living thing is dependent on the continuance of its healthy activity.

WORRY. An English writer of prominence asserts that the majority of people kill themselves by lives of indulgence of mind and body. Mental inactivity is injurious to physical health, and it is rare to find the idler among the list of centenarians. Healthy brain activity is essential to life and justifies the aphorism that "It is not work but worry that kills." That enviable man whom nothing worries is the kind, considerate and patient man whom we occasionally meet in this busy world. The ill-tempered, irritable and pessimistic individual, with deranged digestion and bloated liver, is the man with an unbalanced nervous system, who has simply disregarded the natural law of waste and repair. Many acts of philanthrophy are forever lost in the capriciousness of a disordered liver or a defective digestive apparatus. Worry, grief, passion and fretting are powerful nervous shocks. "There is no sensation," says Tuke, "whether general or special, excited by agents acting on the body from without, which cannot also be excited from within by emotional states affecting the sensory ganglia, such sensation being referred by the mind to the point at which the nerve terminates in the body." The emotional states arrest the function of digestion and impair the bodily functions. Self-control is a powerful palladium against nervous prostration. It is exceptional to find a neurasthenic in individuals who have acquired a knowledge of self government. "Every one can master a grief but he that has it," but we are all competent to construct for ourselves a philosophy of complacency. Such philosophy need not resolve itself into indolence and apathy, nor need it assume the aspects of stoicism. When misfortune or disaster overtakes the Turk he attributes it to the will of God, or more often to fate

(Kismet), and he piously ejaculates: "It is fate" (*Kismet dir*) or "God will provide" (*Allahkerim*). The cultivation of some belief which inculates the doctrines of contentment should be encouraged. It may be a difficult matter to control the emotions, but mastery can be attained by training. I know many neurasthenics who suffer relapses whenever exposed to some intense emotion. When self control is difficult, individuals must avoid conditions which introduce them to such influences. They must avoid going to funerals, reading death notices and newspapers with their daily menu of sensationalism. They should cultivate the companionship of people who may dream of unhappiness but wake up laughing. The worries of some people are often so ridiculous that they must be regarded as the emanations of a diseased mind. I knew one woman, who, after a rest cure for neurasthenia, suffered only one inconvenience, and that was, that she had heard that recovery from a "rest cure" only lasted five years, and at the end of that time she feared she would suffer a relapse. My patient was very much like the woman whose physician asked after her health replied dolefully: "I feel very well; but I always feel bad when I feel well, because I know I am going to feel worse afterwards."

THE ABUSE OF ALCOHOL, COFFEE, TEA, AND TOBACCO.

ALCOHOL, is one of the greatest scourges of the nervous system. Consumed even in the smallest amounts by persons of a nervous temperament it will induce organic changes in the nerve tissues like those of old age. The habitual use of alcohol stands foremost, after heredity, as a single independent cause of insanity. The psychic degeneration of alcoholism is characteristic, and consists of gradually weakening memory and will, slowness of perception and judgment, loss of the moral and esthetic sense, with paroxysms of depression, anger and irritability.   There is no organ of the body which is not implicated in chronic alcoholism, but it is as a *nerve intoxicant* that its most pernicious effects are manifest.   The nervously inclined first become addicted to alcohol in some form believing that it is a stimulant. This is not a fact, for its chief action is depressant and under its influence the actual amount of work that is capable of achievement is less than when it is not taken. The stimulating effects of alcohol are more apparent than real.   By anesthetizing sensation, a temporary release only is secured from the morbid sensations experienced by the neurasthenic.

Morphin and a host of other remedies have a like effect, and it is this fictitious sensation of well-being that is responsible for the prevalence of drug addiction among neurasthenics.   There are many neurasthenics whose symptoms may be directly traced to the alcohol habit.   Such individuals suffer from gastric and nutritional disturbances, mental symptoms and paralysis.

The neurasthenic must be especially warned against the so-called "nerve foods" and other preparations advertised under fascinating names by unscrupulous manufacturers, for many of them contain powerful sedatives, which are merely palliative in their action and ultimately conduce to some pernicious drug habit.

Coffee, Tea and Cocoa.   Caffeine, the active principle of coffee, *theine*, of tea and the alkaloid of cocoa are chemically identical and have the same vicious effects when used inordinately.   Many nervous affections are wholly attributable to their use, in fact, they may duplicate all the symptoms of neurasthenia. Nervous individuals display a definite idiosyncracy toward these substances, hence they should never be employed in such persons.

BODILY DISORDERS. Syphilis is a paradigm of this type of irritants. Here many factors conspire to make the subject a likely victim of neurasthenia. First, there is the mental factor, for there are many persons who once having contracted the disease interpret every bodily derangement as a manifestation of syphilis. Then there is the reduced state of the body induced by injudicious medication, or by the poison of the disease itself, which makes the subject susceptible. Nutritional disturbances provoked by syphilis often make the nervous system the object of least resistance. *Syphilophobia*, or the morbid dread of having contracted syphilis produces intense mental suffering in some individuals and it is also the case when other venereal diseases have, or are supposed to have been acquired. The anxiety of mind conquers the entire being. Sleep, digestion and nutrition are in consequence impaired, and the unending terror may last a lifetime unless controlled by the physician, who is often able by the modern aids of science, to make innocuous the indiscretions arising from venereal disease. Often the sexual madness has no real foundation; a harmless skin eruption, lax, or too lightly drawn testicles, innocent pimples and the like are apt to be construed as manifestations of venereal disease.

INFLUENZA. This affection is likely to be followed by neurasthenia which is sometimes severe, prolonged and obstinate. Other infectious diseases, like malaria and typhoid fever as well as other debilitating diseases are not infrequently followed by neurasthenia, and, indeed, the convalescence of such diseases is made up almost wholly of neurasthenic symptoms.

RAILWAY INJURIES. A nervous condition may follow railway and other injuries, especially when associated with fright. The neurasthenia following such accidents is known as *traumatic neurasthenia*, or "railway spine," and differs in no wise from neurasthenia dependent on other causes.

PHYSIOLOGICAL FACTORS. Puberty in both sexes, and the puerperal state and change of life in women, as well as the tissue changes peculiar to old age (*senility*), are periods in life when the nervous system is subject to excessive strain which increases its vulnerability. Puberty occurs between the thirteenth and twentieth years, a period of life in which remarkable physical and mental changes occur. The evolution of the sexual characters and development of reproduction, give rise to new sensations and strong emotions. The mind, especially of the boy, becomes charged with emotional, sentimental, amatory and fantastic imaginings and vicious habits are formed. In the *puerperal state* pregnancy diminishes the vitality of woman, debilitating and weakening her entire system, thus making her a prey to the many disorders consequent on nervous breakdown.

The *change of life* (menopause), in women between the ages of forty and fifty years, is another epoch fraught with mischief to the nervous system, and it is rare to find in this period of involution, a woman free from nervous manifestations.

The disequilibration associated with the cessation of ovulation and menstruation is a menace to mental integrity.

During the senile period of life, tissue involution is likely to be attended by numerous mental disorders. A conspicuous sign is loss of memory for recent events and the individual's interest becomes centered in his physical comforts and needs.

MORAL CAUSES. It is an axiom, that every time a muscular movement is made, less resistance is made by the nerve center in control of that special motion, and so it is with the moral education of the child, the oftener the latter is permitted to perpetuate a wrong, the easier will its repetition become. Discipline of the child begins at home and attention to their morals is more important than books.—" A man," said Johnson, " is in general better pleased when he has a good dinner upon his table, than when his wife speaks Greek," and a parent would be better pleased if his boy could be taught to escape the dominion of habit by self control than if he knew all the Euclidean axioms. Unfortunately the boy does not know until later in life that self-denial is of more value than indulgence. " Those who would be young when they are old should be old when they are young. Old age in youth should mean parental control.

BRAIN CHANGES IN NEURASTHENIA.

Physiologic experiments demonstrate that in fatigue of the nervous system, the *nerve cells*, which in health are plump, become shrunken and become restored to their original shape and size only after prolonged rest. Brain cells have been compared by a recent writer to small baloons ready for an ascent. When seen under the microscope they are round and full and give evidence of being distended. The cells of the tired brain,

3

on the other hand, are seen to be shrunken, as an air ball or toy baloon, from which most of the air or gas has escaped.

When our brains begin to work after a refreshing rest or sleep they are, continues the same writer, full of nerve fluid, which the absorbents of the body and brain have stored up there like bees fill their comb.   So soon as work begins, this vital force is sapped to meet the demands upon the brain, and the process that goes on during the whole time it is working may be described in the following way:

Imagine that these cells are small goblets filled with liquid, and that they have a tiny stem, through which runs a tube or opening; the liquid in the goblet is drained by the demands of mind and body, and slowly trickles through the opening, drop by drop, until either the work ceases or the goblet is exhausted.

This latter condition is not often reached, for the simple reason that the owner of the brain is very much more likely to collapse.   When the cell has yielded half its vital fluid you begin to experience a feeling of fatigue, and if you go on drawing the contents of the cells you are doing yourself injury in proportionate degree, and nature will make you pay for it in some way or other.

But all the cells are not involved in any kind of mental work, which means that one part of the brain may be very actively at work while the other is resting and storing up nerve fluid.   Thus it is that a man suffering from brain fag may leave his books and go golfing or cycling and feel that he is really resting, other cells are being called upon for work now, while the tired ones, those required for mental activity are enjoying repose.

But it follows that the part of the brain which is called into activity for bodily exercise is now getting tired, while the other part of the brain is still at work to some extent, and so the whole of our brain cells become fatigued, and total rest, in the shape of sleep, is absolutely essential.

The " neuron theory " of Hodge,[4] is of special interest in determining the pathology of neurasthenia. Hodge studied the nerve cells of swallows, pigeons and bees before and after fatigue and in all cases he observed noteworthy changes. After rest, the cells were large and plump, well defined and the nuclei easily demonstrated. After a day's flight, the cells became small, the nuclei indistinct, the protoplasm granular and shrunken and the cell processes striated. Dercum claims, that in chronic cases of neurasthenia, the blood contains toxic substances derived from the excessive waste of nerve tissue ; and Mosso, who injected the blood of a fatigued animal into one at rest, obtained in the latter the characteristic signs of fatigue. The conclusion that may be formulated as the result of the preceding observations is practically as follows :

FATIGUE NEURASTHENIA. There is a *neurasthenia dependent on overwork* or over-functioning, a form correctly specified by Savill,[5] as " fatigue-neurasthenia " which is dependent on exhaustion of the nerve cells. The latter which may be aptly compared to electric cells furnish a definite amount of electricity, but after continuous use without intermission, they exhaust themselves, and their output of electricity, an expression of their function, becomes diminished and the mechanism of the organs can no longer be put in motion, or, if so, with great difficulty. Rest will restore the storage capacity of the nerve cells as it will the

electric cells.   There is the law of Edinger which is
quite apposite in relation to neurasthenia, viz: increased function, if regularly and gradually increased
leads first of all to increas growth; if carried to excess
however, or is irregular and spasmodic, it leads to
waste and degeneration of the tissues concerned.

Every function of the body is controlled and operated
by the nervous system.   The latter which dominates
the functions of the mind likewise controls the action
of the muscles.   We haven't two nervous systems nor
two brains and it is this mistaken conception of the
functions of the nervous system which has made con-
firmed neurasthenics out of individuals who have ex-
pended too much nerve force in excessive muscular
development under the supposition that they were developing their minds.   If the theory of muscularity
were correct, intellectual giants would be recruited
from dray horses and pugilists.

SUMMARY.

1. The chief symptom of neurasthenia is tire. Without the latter sign, the disease cannot be said to exist.

2. While neurasthenia occurs most frequently between the ages of twenty and fifty, it may occur during other periods of life. Children are by no means exempt and, if the affection in the child is unrecognized, it is because the nervous system of the child reacts differently to the exciting causes than does the same system in the adult, and for the additional reason, that the mind in the child is eliminated from participation in the physical symptoms.

3. Nerve force, has been compared to electricity, but this comparison does not improve our conception of the nature of nerve force, which like electricity is very obscure. The comparison will aid the neurologist in framing a positive knowledge concerning the action and laws that govern nerve force, which in relation to electricity are precise and extensive.

4. Muscularity is not essential to intellectual development, on the contrary physical overwork drains our capital of nerve force and disturbs the equilibrium of mental and physical health. The "mens sana in corpore sano" can only be attained by a judicious exercise of both mind and body.

5. Nerve health is a condition subject to the discretion of the individual: it is the resultant of the income and expenditure of nerve force.

6. Stimulants, like drugs used for the relief of nervousness, have been invented for both the patient and physician. They relieve the former of obeying the laws of hygiene and the latter of inculcating them.

They assist in the early death of foolish neurasthenics so that their fellow sufferers may learn the correct path to health.

7. " They who would be young when they are old, must be old when they are young." Everything which promotes the general health will promote recovery from neurasthenia, for anything which will influence health will have a corresponding effect on *health*.

8. That " An idle brain is the devil's workshop," is never better illustrated than in an insane hospital."

9. In studying the relation which exists between venereal and nervous diseases, we note the will of omniscient Providence dedicating to virtue, vigorous manhood and a noble life. When a staid and respected member of society, developes in later years a post-venereal disease, the picture he presents, is that of respectability painted on a back-ground of vice.

10. Neurasthenia has no definite pathology and all hypotheses which hint in that direction have not exceeded the realms of theory. We recognize the disease as we do the physical forces by their effects, viz: an acute or chronic functional nervous trouble manifested by nervous weakness and irritability, in which the patient is easily exhausted and is acutely responsive to trivial irritations.

11. Self-culture embraces a training of the physical, moral and intellectual parts of man. All must be equally and judiciously trained. An exclusive training of the physical part will develop an athlete; of the moral, an enthusiast ; of the intellectual, a crank.

CHAPTER III.

SPECIAL IRRITANTS OF NEURASTHENIA.

THE PRIMARY FACTOR IN NEURASTHENIA.—SEXUAL NEUR-
ASTHENIA.—CONGESTIVE NEURASTHENIA.—URIC ACID
NEURASTHENIA.—AUTO-TOXEMIC NEURASTHENIA.—AB-
DOMINAL NEURASTHENIA.—DYSPEPSIA AND NEURAS-
THENIA.—SPLANCHNIC NEURASTHENIA.

In the preceding chapter, the cause of neurasthenia
was attributed in brief to *overstrain* of the nervous
system provoked by the various mental, moral and
physical causes, the result, as Beard puts it of *over-
civilization*. Very soon investigators sought to explain how this irritability and weakness of the nerve
cells was brought about. Medical writers are being
rapidly weaned from the doctrine that an hereditarily
degenerate nervous system is the primary factor in
neurasthenia. The assumption of such an hypothesis
would mean the relegation of personal responsibility to
heredity and would grant immunity to the transgressor.
The fact is, that a number of neurasthenics owe their
infirmity to indiscretions, and a still larger class to
morbid organic functions, which, if corrected, would
cure their disease.

Charcot claimed that the working-classes were not
exempt from neurasthenia; on the contrary, physical

39

fatigue, poverty and the constant anxiety to make both ends meet were as potent in inducing neuras-thenia as the brain work of professional or business men.

Physicians now recognize that certain predisposing influences exist to induce neurasthenia, even though an inherent weakness of the nervous system can be ex-cluded.

As a result of this recognition, reference is now made to special forms of neurasthenia which will en-gage our attention.   '

Many affections which have hitherto been recognized as diseases by themselves are either symptomatic of neurasthenia or induce the latter affection by their persistency.

SEXUAL NEURASTHENIA.   In their monograph on Sexual Neurasthenia,[6] Beard and Rockwell, refer to the various maladies of the male sexual appara-tus, viz; impotence, spermatorrhoea, prostatorrhea, irritable prostate, etc., as mere manifestations of neurasthenia. The trend of modern opinion is not only to regard sexual ailments as manifestations of neurasthenia, but as the cause of the affection. Again, the state which sexual disorders induce is not neces-sarily a neurasthenic one. Witness as an instance the masturbator. His condition is one of mental de-pression with disinclination to work and study. He is nervous and irritable : numb feelings are felt in the hands and feet, etc. His physiognomy is character-istic and by no means tallies with that of neurasthenia, viz : pale complexion, furtive eye, dilated pupil, restless and depressed appearance, moist and flabby palms, etc. In women, masturbation is a frequent cause of hysteroepilepsy. Freud [7] avers that neurasthenia can always be traced to excessive masturbation, unnatural sexual intercourse, unsatisfied impulses, abstinency with inflamed desires, interrupted coitus, etc., and he urges the physician to assume an abnormal sexual life as his guiding star in the causation of neurasthenia.

Hottinger [8] contends that many functional derangements of the genito-urinary system, which have been referred to as symptoms of neurasthenia, have as their basis some form of prostatitis, and that the so-called neurasthenia disappears when the prostatitis is cured.   Fuller [9] refers neurasthenia to a seminal vesiculitis; Ravogli to a chronic urethritis and syphilis; and Eastman [10] to impaired sexual gratification, laceration of the perineum, etc. in women.   The foregoing writers are unquestionably extreme in their views, but their observations convey a modicum of truth if for no other reason than to emphasize that a local source of irritation may be responsible if not for neurasthenia, at least for neurasthenic symptoms.

CONGESTIVE NEURASTHENIA.   Whittle, of London, in 1889, wrote an interesting brochure on this special form of neurasthenia, but it seems to have escaped the serious consideration of the medical profession.   I have repeatedly been able to confirm the observations of Whittle.   He describes a form of nerve depression resulting from brain congestion and illustrates the remarkable efficacy of bloodletting, either by leeches or venesection, in its treatment.   The particular patients, who are thus benefited, look to the uninitiated eye, the picture of health, but are really miserable victims to whom actual pain or some evident disease would prove an agreeable distraction.   Their faces are flushed, eyes watery and there is a lightness in the head with occasional aching of a dull, heavy character about the forehead.   The majority of cases occur between the ages of thirty and forty, very few under twenty-five or over fifty.   This includes the most active and wearing period of life.   If a man can stand the strain of this period, he will be proof against anything he may encounter afterward.   Congestive neurasthenia occurs more frequently in males than females and the most constant factor in its production is continuous brain strain.

During sleep, such as it is, the body rests but not the brain.   As a result the brain becomes unduly charged with blood, leading to congestion, which nothing seems to relieve so quickly and marvelously as blood-letting.   Leeching is one of the good remedies out of fashion, and while formerly it was the custom to bleed too much, it is unfortunate that now we do not bleed enough.   I remember one congestive neurasthenic who, by actual calculation, had consulted twenty-three different physicians, among whom were some of the leading nerve specialists of Europe.   In addition he had made a number of sea voyages and visited many celebrated spas but with absolutely no relief.   Incidentally an eye trouble necessitated the application of leeches by his oculist to the temples, resulting in immediate relief to his nerve symptoms which had hitherto baffled all treatment.   Six months later his old symptoms returned but the reapplication of leeches and the withdrawal of blood from the brain vessels was as successful as in the primary instance.

URIC ACID NEURASTHENIA.   Brain workers often suffer from a series of perplexing symptoms which baffle the skill of their medical advisers.   Such sufferers are usually good livers and lead sedentary lives.   With such, insomnia, headache, mental depression, backache, and dyspepsia are prominent signs.

When Alexander Haig, of London, issued his work, " Uric acid as a factor in the causation of disease," he attempted to make many problems clear which had heretofore remained unrecognized. His uric acid theory is briefly as follows : Uric acid occurs in the blood in traces during health. It is derived chiefly from foods, and persons who eat an excess of food and take little exercise, produce an excessive quantity of uric acid, which, accumulating in the blood, gives rise to a train of symptoms. The blood being naturally alkaline, holds the uric acid in solution, but, if from any cause, the blood becomes acid, it can no longer hold the uric acid in solution and consequently the latter is precipitated. Now, the joints, muscles and ligaments are favorable sites for the precipitation of uric acid, hence those who suffer from uric acid poisoning complain of muscular pains in the back and joint stiffness. This theory, while primarily fascinating, soon became the subject of critical analysis with results inimical to its tenability. It was shown that uric acid was absolutely non-irritating to the tissues and could be injected in large amounts into animals, as well as administered in their food with no toxic results whatever, in other words, *uric acid itself does not produce* disease.

It is not the retention of uric acid in the system which produces the so-called *uric acid diathesis* but the presence of certain products, the result of deficient oxidation. These products are known as the purin or alloxuric bases, like xanthin, guanin, adenin, etc. They are highly toxic, and are normally burned in the body through the process of oxidation and are finally converted and eliminated as uric acid, a very harmless product. The toxic substances in question are derived

in part from food and in part from the worn out body
cells.

Woods-Hutchinson[11] clearly defines our present status
regarding the uric acid theory in referring to the nature
and causation of gout, viz: "A toxemia of varying
causation, usually of gastro-intestinal origin, accompanied by the formation of an excess of urates, this
excess of urates being due to the breaking down of the
leucocytes and fixed cells in the attempt to neutralise
the poison—in other words, being the measure of the resisting power of the body tissues. The formation and
introduction of the toxins, be it well understood, are
by no means confined to the gouty; it is only the
nature of the resistance of the body to them that gives
the character of gout."

This carries us to a consideration of *gastro-intestinal
diseases* as a cause of neurasthenia, which I will include
under the caption of *Auto-toxemic neurasthenia.*

AUTO-TOXEMIC NEURASTHENIA. In general, auto-toxemia refers to poisoning of the organism superinduced
by poisons generated within that organism, a condition,
in other words, of self infection. Self-infection may
occur from the following causes: 1. Retention in the
body of certain substances destined for excretion (*Auto-
intoxication of retention*).

2. Absorption of substances from normal or abnormal cavities of the body developed from putrefaction or fermentation (Auto-intoxication of resorption).

3. Substances developed from disturbances in the
cells and secretions of organs (histogenic auto-intoxication).

4. Poisoning, the result of toxine absorption developed by micro-parasites (auto-intoxication of infection).

The second variety of auto-intoxication of which re-

sorption from the gastro-intestinal canal is the most conspicuous example and which is best understood will occupy our attention.

GASTRO-INTESTINAL AUTO-INTOXICATION.—Bouchard [12] was one of the first to show that man is constantly standing, as it were, on the brink of a precipice. Every moment of his life, he runs the risk of being overpowered by poisons generated within his system. The healthy and unhealthy body is a receptacle and laboratory of poisons. Self poisoning is only inhibited by the activity of the skin, kidneys and bowels. These poisons are normally manufactured in our gastro-intestinal canal, and were it not for the action of the bowels, kidneys and skin, many of us would succumb to auto-intoxication. Aside from the excretory organs which promote the excretion of the poisons, the alimentary canal and the liver are endowed with functions capable of rendering innocuous many of the toxic substances.

The proponents of this theory maintain that in health, auto-intoxication does not occur, either because sufficient of the toxic material is not absorbed and is rapidly excreted, or if absorbed, the poisons are made inert by the action of the liver, blood and tissue cells. On the other hand, self infection occurs in disease of the gastro-intestinal mucous membrane which facilitates the entrance into the blood of the toxic substances, or because the liver and the tissue cells are incapable of making them innocuous.

The symptoms of auto-intoxication are difficult of enumeration, simply because the recognition of the affection itself is difficult.

Observation however has taught us, that the toxic products are capable of producing local symptoms, viz: various digestive disturbances and general disturbances of the nervous system. Such signs may duplicate the symptomatic picture of neurasthenia with profound depression, mental disturbances, epilepsy, locomotor ataxia and mental exaltation. This varying symptomatic picture depends on the nature of the toxic substances absorbed, some exciting, others depressing the nervous system. Schroeder von der Kolk, some years ago, demonstrated that acute, confusional insanity was associated with fecal accumulation in the colon.

As already stated, it is difficult to associate many of the symptoms with gastro-intestinal poisoning and here the results of treatment could offer us some assistance. In a few instances, we know that manifold nervous symptoms have subsided after free evacuation of the bowels, but in my own observations, where there was every reason to suspect intestinal auto-toxemia, the results of treatment were quite unsatisfactory.

The treatment in question was that which is conceded to be the best for intestinal auto-toxemia: 1. An exclusively milk diet which reduces to a minimum the introduction of poisonous food products. 2. Daily irrigation of the stomach and bowels. 3. Purgatives. 4. Intestinal antiseptics. I am constrained to conclude, that the auto-intoxication theory, while of great scientific value and hints at many possibilities in the future is not sufficiently developed at the present time to prove of much practical value to the neurasthenic.

ABDOMINAL NEURASTHENIA. There are a number of abdominal affections which have been cited as causes of neurasthenia, and I have grouped them all under the caption of *abdominal neurasthenia*. The belief that the abdominal cavity was responsible for many diseases, notably, hypochondriasis is of ancient origin.

The term hypochondriasis, originated from the supposition that its cause was resident in the hypochondriac region, owing to the feelings of distress and uneasiness which prevailed there. Broussais (1772–1838) advocated, as his most powerful treatment, the application of leeches to the abdomen and as many as thirty to fifty were applied at a single seance. This was hirudinomania with a vengeance. In 1785, Johann Kamp, published a work, entitled, "For physicians and patients, a new method for the radical cure of pernicious diseases, specially hypochondriasis, which have their origin in the abdomen." He refers to many nervous diseases which were unquestionably of abdominal origin, and his treatment consisted in the main of enemas made from decoctions of herbs.

Voetsch, in 1874, published his work on "coprostasis" (hardened fecal matter in the intestines), and recites in detail the histories of fifty-eight patients with manifold disturbances in different organs that were directly attributed to habitual constipation.

In 1885, Glénard issued an important work, in which he attributed neurasthenia to *enteroptosis*, a condition in which there was a prolapse of one or other of the abdominal organs. The symptoms described by him and known as Glénard's disease occurred in the following order of succession: 1. Debility and lassitude. 2. Sensations of uneasiness, weight, dragging, craving, emptiness, etc., in the abdomen. 3. Symptoms of dyspepsia. 4. Nervous symptoms. The researches of Glénard were of great importance, but subsequent observers did not confirm his conclusions in their entirety. The conservative opinion now is, that prolapse of the abdominal organs may occur without neurasthenic symptoms and that neurasthenia may occur without gastric symptoms.

Dunin,[13] in 1891, demonstrated that habitual constipation is associated with a train of neurasthenic symptoms, but he cautions, and in my experience wisely, against the regular employment of purgatives which only aggravate the symptoms.

Federn,[14] in 1894, published a monograph, in which he attempted to show, that nervous symptoms (neurasthenia), contrary to accepted doctrines, are by no means dependent on a nervous system faulty by heredity, but that they are caused primarily by intestinal disturbances. The latter cause an increase in the blood pressure and to this must be attributed the nervous symptoms. In this increased blood pressure, he argues, there is a mechanic irritation of the tissues and organs, for when the blood pressure is reduced to normal all nervous manifestations cease. In the majority of neurasthenics, there is a partial intestinal atony with or without constipation or intestinal catarrh.

DYSPEPSIA AND NEURASTHENIA. Most writers admit that dyspepsia is frequently an associated condition of neurasthenia, but its definite relation to the disease in question is a matter of doubt. Some maintain that neurasthenia may produce a particular kind of stomach disturbance, others, that if stomach disturbances develop they are merely manifestations of a neurasthenic condition. The latter view is based on the principle, that in health all the organs work harmoniously: One is dependent on the other for the normal performance of its work. If one suffers they all suffer, a vicious circle being thereby established.

Some one organ, however, it may be the stomach, heart or liver, usually bears the brunt of nervous exhaustion. Why this is so, is difficult to say, other than by supposing that every person like Achilles has some vulnerable spot. Some persons when they have a "nerve storm," center all their abnormal sensations in the heart, others in the stomach, others in the head.

Still others contend that neurasthenia in a certain proportion of cases is the result of the gastric disorder. The latter contention is, however, difficult of definite solution. Those who support the latter theory, notably Savill,[15] claim that dyspeptic disturbances often precede the symptoms of neurasthenia and ergo neurasthenia may be provoked by dyspepsia. Who can tell, however, if the dyspeptic disturbances were not the initial symptoms of neurasthenia? This much is true, however, that gastric derangements, in fact all abdominal affections complicating neurasthenia are attended by depression of spirits, circulatory, and many vague nervous disturbances; nutrition is seriously embarassed and there is a decided falling off in weight.

How a digestive disturbance operates is a matter of conjecture only. There is necessarily a defective nutrition of the nerve apparatus and there is also an increased elaboration of toxic products. I believe that many cases of neurasthenia and I wish particularly to be understood in my contention, *not all cases*, have an abdominal origin: that in many cases, whatever the nature of the ailment, the neurasthenia may be referred to a defect in the nerve apparatus which controls the supply of blood in the abdominal cavity, and furthermore, that the condition is eradicable by the adoption of certain simple methods based on scientific principles. The form of neurasthenia in question, I will call *splanchnic neurasthenia*, which will be the subject of discussion in succeeding chapters.

4

SUMMARY.

1. A congenital degenerate nervous system is not the primary factor in neurasthenia, although such a system will react more easily to irritants which produce the disease.

2. Deranged bodily functions are often responsible for the neurasthenic state, and their recognition demands unusual diagnostic acumen on the part of the physician. The latter will heed the trite remarks of Sir William Savory : "Consciousness of one's ignorance may do much to avert the errors of carelessness, and he who has confidence in his own judgment should of all men be most careful in inquiry."

3. The uric acid theory of neurasthenia is most fascinating but faulty, and even the latter could be condoned were definite results achieved by treatment executed in accordance with the theory. The patient is not a theoretician but an utilitarian. He visits his physician with a definite object in view, to get well, and mere theories will not influence him. The uric acid theory, it must be conceded, at least inculcates the doctrine of moderation in eating and selection of food, a doctrine which is most salutary in all diseases.

4. The theory of gastro-intestinal auto-intoxication, while endowed with a modicum of truth, is in a practical sense undeveloped and furnishes no definite clue to the symptoms of self-poisoning nor to its treatment.

5. Gastro-intestinal disturbances, of whatever nature, seriously compromise the integrity of the nervous system, either by inducing neurasthenia or aggravating it if it exists,

6. There is a form of nervousness which I have designated as splanchnic neurasthenia, which is capable of cure, and the treatment is based on definite scientific principles.

This special form of neurasthenia has heretofore escaped recognition.

CHAPTER IV.

THE GENERAL AND SPECIAL SYMPTOMS OF NEURAS-
THENIA.

MOTOR DISORDERS.—SENSORY DISTURBANCES.— EYE SIGNS—
EAR SIGNS.—BRAIN SIGNS.— HEART SIGNS AND THE PULSE.—
PULMONARY ANEMIA. — STOMACH AND INTESTINAL SIGNS.—
SEXUAL SIGNS.—FORMS OF NEURASTHENIA.— DIAGNOSIS
AND PROGNOSIS OF NEURASTHENIA.

THE GENERAL SYMPTOMS. These may be divided
into: 1. Motor disorders. 2. Sensory disturbances.
3. Disturbances of the special senses.

MOTOR DISORDERS. *Muscular fatigue* is a constant
sign. Muscular contraction is excited through the
nervous system by nerve impulses which reach the
fibres of the muscle. Such contractions may be voluntary, automatic or reflex, but, in all instances, they
predicate a discharge of nerve force from a nerve
center. When a muscle contracts it transforms an
equivalent amount of energy. The latter consists in
oxidizing food substances contained in its fibers or
burning them at a relatively low temperature. The
chief food-substances consumed by a contracting muscle
are glucose or grape sugar, glycogen and fat. Fatigue
of muscle is essentially caused by the consumption of
material necessary for contraction and the storing up
in the muscle of waste products produced by its own

activity. Some people naturally tire more easily than others owing to the fact that the waste products responsible for the fatigue in the one are less easily removed or accumulate more readily. Massage of the muscles rapidly removes the evidence of fatigue, simply because the waste products from the muscles are washed away into the circulation by this maneuver. The fatigue in neurasthenia probably has its origin in the nervous system and only indirectly in the muscles; for, if we pursue the same argument which physiologists accept as the cause of muscular fatigue, viz: the accumulation of waste substances, it is reasonable to assume, that a like condition prevails in the nervous system. If one tests the strength of the muscles in neurasthenia by means of the dynamometer, while the muscles may show a diminished response, it is by no means proportionate to the diminished vigor experienced by the patient.

Marcet,[16] has shown that the time during which an individual can sustain a voluntary muscle contraction is determined by the endurance of the brain centers engaged in the act of volition, rather than by that of the muscles themselves. The very moment these centers are exhausted the muscle contraction gives way. Another fact developed by the same writer, and as it seems to me, an important one which can be applied to neurasthenia is, that volition can be fatigued when exerted in imagination as well as in actual muscle effort.

Muscular tire in the neurasthenic is expressed by general muscular weakness, lack of endurance, a tired feeling, a feeling of never being rested and a sensation of extreme weariness on rising in the morning. In severe cases, patients remain in bed for indefinite periods, having assured themselves by aid of their morbid imagination that they are incapable of any kind of muscular effort. When fatigue symptoms become exaggerated, they become painful and are described by the patient as aches.

TREMOR. This is often brought out by the slightest muscular effort and Lemarcq, found it present in eighty-five per cent. of neurasthenics. The tremor is a fine one and present most often in the hands, but may be general, including the knees, legs and the closed eyelids. In pronounced cases, the fine tremor may be substituted by twitching of the muscles, and they may become so pronounced in the face and tongue, that on seeing such individuals for the first time, one is constrained to think of general paresis. All the *reflexes* are exaggerated.

SENSORY DISTURBANCES.—*Headache* is a common sign. It may be constantly present or evoked by any mental or muscular effort or some emotion. In most instances, the headache is not really described as an ache, but a feeling of heavy weight or constriction about the head. Some describe the sensation of a closely fitting lead cap on the head. Charcot described the head-sensation as the "casque neurasthenique," a feeling as though the patient were wearing a tight-fitting helmet. The head sensation may be also described by the patient as a feeling of pressure or ache in definite regions, notably the base of the brain, the top or front of the head or at the temples. Still others experience a heaviness or throbbing and a sensation as if wind or water were running under the scalp. The neurasthenic head sensations usually occur when the patient wakes up and last during the day to disappear on retiring.

BACKACHE, or a sensation of weariness, is a frequent symptom and the older writers referred to this
symptom as "spinal irritation."

If the signs of so called "spinal irritation" are pronounced, the feeling of intense weariness prevents the
patient from sitting or standing for any length of time.
Women suffer more frequently than men from the back
sensations, and a favorite location for the tenderness
in women is at the extreme end of the spine (Coccyg-
odynia)

All cases of backache are not necessarily of neurasthenic origin but are often due to a *faulty spinal
attitude*. Thus the attitude of children with "round
shoulders" will substitute ligamentous for muscular
support. Deformities of the foot, like flat foot, will
conduce to pain in the back owing to the faulty attitude assumed by such persons.

PAINS IN THE LIMBS. These are sensations variously described as hot flushes, tingling, cold, numbness,
stiffness, soreness, etc., in any and all parts of the
body. In some instances, the pains become fixed in
some definite region, as over the heart or stomach, a
condition described by Blocq as "topoalgia" or local
neurasthenia.[17]

SPECIAL SYMPTOMS.

EYE SIGNS. Vision is never seriously affected. An
early sign is a blurring of the vision on using the eyes
for any length of time and which may become so pronounced that the patient is unable to perform any
work requiring the use of the eyes for any length of
time. Often the vision becomes veiled and things
look strange and unreal. Patients often complain

of a defect in visual memory, i.e., they see some familiar object, it may be a person or a thing, but they do not remember it with their normal facility. It must be conceded, in the light of modern observation, that there are cases of neurasthenia, may I call them "ocular neurasthenias," which owe their origin solely to some easily remedied eye defect. Such defect may be due to an error in refraction or to defects in the ocular muscles.

The remote effects of *eye strain* may include not only neurasthenia but vertigo, migraine, chorea, and epilepsy. The refractive condition of the eye is rarely normal, and no muscles of the body are subjected to such excessive strain as the ocular muscles. If one wishes to appreciate the effects of eye strain, all that is necessary is to wear for a few minutes the glasses of another person suffering from astigmatism. In the recognition of an ocular defect, the task of the physician is by no means ended. He must determine whether the eye-defect is alone responsible for the symptoms or whether they are aggravated by other conditions, as defective hygiene, bad habits, etc.; he must treat the nervous system after correction of the ocular defect, and he must direct the patient to an oculist and not an optician. Even all oculists are not specially skilled in correcting errors of refraction and many relegate this important matter to assistants or execute it in a perfunctory manner.

Drooping of the lids, inequality of the pupils or excessive mobility of the iris are symptoms which have been observed in neurasthenia. It has been noted in testing the visual field in neurasthenia, that when an object is brought from without into and across the field of vision that it is seen in wider range than when it is placed in the center of vision and carried gradually outward toward the periphery. This is known as "*Foerster's shifting type*," and is the reverse of the normal condition.

EAR SIGNS. Abnormal ringing, singing, whistling and roaring sounds may be heard although hearing may be intact.

As a rule, these signs are associated with some actual disease of the middle ear, in elderly people, with degenerative changes in the blood vessels, and in young persons, with some abnormal state of the blood. Hearing in neurasthenics is often hyperesthetic and they show excessive sensibility to noises, the slightest noise startles them. Even melodious music is borne with intolerance.

BRAIN SIGNS. The capacity for *mental work* becomes diminished. Any mental effort is attended by a sense of fatigue and distress. Fixing the attention on anything is deficient and often impossible, and the ability to originate ideas or to think intelligently or connectedly becomes lessened, or is abolished entirely. There is lack of *will power*, and this deficiency is frequently expressed by vacillation or indecision. *Mental irritability* is another sign added to the cerebral manifestations. The patient becomes annoyed at little things which before failed to disturb his equilibrium. There is loss of *memory*. Ideas do not occur with the usual vigor and patients affirm that "they cannot think straight." The fear of insanity is common. Attracted by their symptoms, they become introspective, misconstrue their sensations and develop *phobias* or morbid fears. *Morbid fears* rarely become insane delusions. Fear in neurasthenics develops as a result of weakness or loss of courage.

Some fear to be alone, some fear darkness, others narrow or high places, others crowds and still others an open space, etc. Some fear dirt or infection by disease. A neurasthenic recognizes the absurdity of his fears and is able to dispel them, whereas the hypochondriac regards such fears as actual conditions and cannot be convinced to the contrary.

Morbid fears are technically described as follows:

1. *Pathophobia*, fear of disease.
2. *Claustrophobia*, fear of narrow spaces.
3. *Photophobia*, fear of light.
5. *Mysophobia*, fear of defilement.

Imperative conceptions and *morbid impulses* are not unknown conditions in neurasthenia. The former refer to ideas which the patient knows are absurd, but which nevertheless occur to him and dominate his thoughts, and often direct his actions. When he is unable to recognize the absurdity of his conception, it becomes a delusion.

A MORBID IMPULSE is an irresistible desire to commit an act which the patient knows to be wrong.

DIMINISHED AFFECTION for those dear to him is another sign which often distresses the patient. Esquirol observes that, "moral alienation is the first step to madness." The patient becomes irritable, fault-finding and resentful. He dreads meeting acquaintances or people. He approaches his daily task with a sense of weariness. He becomes emotional and lachrymose on the slightest pretext. He recounts the history of his illness to every one who will listen and often seems to delight in so doing. As a rule, he regards the future with distrust. His feeling of *mental depression* pictures all sorts of horrible things. He fears that he will never get well or that he will become insane or paralyzed. He cannot bear to read the morning papers lest some accident, or murder or sudden death may distress him.

SLEEPLESSNESS is one of the earliest signs. Sometimes there is difficulty in falling asleep, or the sleep is constantly disturbed. Occasionally the sleep is sound and deep, yet the patient awakens in the morning unrefreshed and often feels more depressed than upon retiring. On closing the eyes in bed, there is, at times, sudden jerking of the legs, or a feeling as of falling. When dreams disturb the sleep, they indicate that the latter is not sound, but partial. In dreams, the brain is in part awake; the will is dormant and the imagination runs riot with incongruous and fantastic images. When many brain centers are active, dreams are consistent and coherent, while, when few centers are working, they are unreal and extravagant. Dreams are evidence of unsound sleep. The dreaming period, in health, rarely occurs until the time for awakening approaches. If the dreaming period comes on early, there is some disorder present in the body which retards the complete rest of the brain. Attempts have been made to classify dreams, but such classifications, from a psychologic standpoint, are purely arbitrary.

RESTLESSNESS is a frequent symptom. The patients keep continually moving and are always "on the fidget." If they are in one place, they want to be somewhere else, in fact, they really do not know what they do want.

VERTIGO or a feeling of dizziness or faintness is not an unusual symptom. It is a disturbance of consciousness, manifested by apparent movement of external objects, or of the subject himself. If the person

himself appears to move, it is known as *subjective*, and
if objects move as *objective vertigo*.

Vertigo experienced when reclining, and disappearing
on rising, is known as *horizontal vertigo*.

The attacks are usually subjective, short in duration
and unaccompanied by nausea. While the sensation is
usually experienced while the patient is up and about,
some persons feel the sensation while in bed as though
they were sinking through it. Vertigo is a cause for
alarm in many patients. There is another form of vertigo occurring in neurasthenics, which is essentially
psychogenetic. It is a sudden sensation of insecurity,
a fear of falling or loss of consciousness. In such instances there is never any real vertigo, nor do the patients fall or lose consciousness, and the condition is
essentially a mental disease. Vertigo is occasioned by
such a multitude of conditions that a diagnosis of " neurasthenic vertigo " is never warranted until other
conditions which are apt to cause it are carefully
excluded.

HEART SIGNS. *Heart Palpitation* is a frequent
symptom.

Palpitation means that the patient is conscious of his
heart's action. A conscious knowledge of any organ
constitutes disease of that organ, not necessarily organic, but more often functional disease. A person
with a healthy heart is not conscious that he has such
an organ. In the mild forms of palpitation only a
fluttering or sinking feeling is experienced. In the
more severe forms, the heart beats violently against
the chest, the arteries throb and the action of the
heart is increased as many times as 150 pulsations per
minute. In nervous palpitation, the face becomes
flushed, and after the attacks large quantities of urine

are passed. An attack may last only a few minutes
or may continue for hours. Palpitation is most often
caused by some digestive disturbance or may result
from emotions or prolonged muscular or mental efforts.

"Rumpf's symptom," is sometimes present. It
consists of making pressure over some painful point in
the body which will bring up the pulse from 80 to 90
to over 100, and it will remain there for one or two
minutes. The heart may be unusually rapid in action
(*heart hurry*), slow, irregular or intermittent. There
may be pains localized in the heart region which radiate down the arms (*false angina pectoris*). Cardiac
disturbances are most frequent in women, in young
persons and in those addicted to the inordinate use of
tobacco, tea, coffee and alcohol. In many neurasthenics, the heart gives unquestionable evidence of weakness, and this is a factor which must be taken into
serious consideration in the treatment of the patient.

THE PULSE. Various attempts have recently been
made by clinicians to endow the pulse in neurasthenia
with certain characteristics, but thus far all efforts in
this direction have been practically futile. My studies
in arterial tension in this disease show that the pulse
is more often of low than high tension, and when the
latter exists it is found in full blooded individuals, in
whom some form of intoxication may be surmised.
Erben,[18] after studying a large number of neurasthenics observed that the customary increase in the pulse
rapidity that follows the movements of the body did
not take place if the patient bent far forward, or, as
Ortner pointed out, if they bend their heads backward.
After either posture, it was observed that the pulse,
after continuing its rhythm for from four to fifteen
beats, there was a sudden retardation of the pulse,

which continued for about sixteen beats, after which the pulse gradually attained its former rapidity.

VASOMOTOR DISTURBANCES. When the vasomotor center is weakened or irritable, flushing and pallor of the skin occur at irregular intervals, specially in women, with cold hands and feet, throbbing noises or fullness in the head, spots before the eyes, dizziness, etc.

THE URINE. This is usually normal, but, after a "nerve storm," it is passed in large quantities, of a pale color and of low specific gravity. *Phosphates* may be present in excess as well as *indican* or *oxalate of lime*, when the case is one of sexual neurasthenia.

THE TEMPERATURE is usually normal, even though the patients experience flushing or burning cutaneous sensations.

THE BLOOD is usually normal, although there are neurasthenics, specially women and young girls, who show an anemic condition of the blood. I have show elsewhere [19] that anemia is often associated with insufficient lung development, a form of anemia which I have designated as *pulmonary anemia.* * In this anemia of pulmonary origin there is not necessarily a diminished number of red blood corpuscles nor of hemoglobin, the element lacking being oxygen (*Anoxemia*). Individuals, the subject of anoxemia, resist all the conventional forms of treatment, but when treated by aid of respiratory exercises to achieve lung development, the anemia disappears. Much benefit is derived from respiratory exercises in the treatment of neurasthenia, and the improvement noted proceeds commensurately with the oxygen-carrying capacity of the blood coloring matter. Other factors may have been at work in improving the nervous symptoms, for we know that

* Appendix, note 1.

healthy lung ventilation means an increased flow of blood and lymph in the nervous system, and this means an augmented supply of oxygen, improved nutrition and removal of waste products.

Stomach Signs. The more I observe dyspeptics, the more certain is my conviction that nervousness is responsible for the majority of cases. We are a nation of dyspeptics, owing to our ceaseless and intense living methods. Repair is not commensurate with waste, and there comes a time to many of us when our functions must suffer. All the organs of the body in health work harmoniously; one is dependent on the other for the normal performance of its work. If one suffers, they all suffer, yet some one organ, it may be the heart, the stomach or the liver, usually bears the brunt of nerve exhaustion.

Nervous indigestion is a frequent complication of nerve strain. The appetite may be unimpaired and even voracious. At other times, the mere thought of food is repugnant. Often the food eaten lies like a heavy weight. The patient belches and is apt to bring up a sour fluid, giving rise to heartburn. The tongue may be perfectly clean throughout the disturbances of digestion. The day has waned when the physician, after casting a furtive glance at the tongue, feeling the pulse and asking a few desultory questions about the stomach, proceeds to prescribe what has been facetiously called a "shotgun" prescription; embodying pepsin and acid to increase digestion, an alkali to correct acidity, a tonic to promote digestion and a purgative to move the bowels. Such a prescription is as much a contradiction as the "whiskey cocktail" described by the perturbed Frenchman, "a little whiskey to make it strong, a little water to make it weak, a little lemon to make it sour, a little sugar to make it sweet, and then you say, here's to you, and you drink it yourself." The scientific physician of to-day takes nothing for granted; he places the patient on a "test meal," after which, he withdraws the contents of the stomach and subjects it to chemic analysis. Having ascertained the ingredients of the gastric juice, he is ready to fulfill his duties as an up-to-date practitioner, and prescribe accordingly. In the majority of cases of nervous dyspepsia, chemic analysis shows no anomaly, and digestion is found to have been completed within the normal time limit. The latter facts are alone characteristic of nervous dyspepsia. Were the digestive trouble of a nature other than nervous, there would be decided changes in the gastric juice, and in the character of the digestion. Nervous dyspeptics instinctively discover that it is not wise to eat too much when nervous or excited, for it is at such a time that gastric signs predominate.

INTESTINAL SIGNS. The chief sign is constipation. Torpidity of the bowels may run in families. Sedentary habits, coupled with excessive eating and a disregard to the call of nature, as well as the character of the food eaten, are common causes of constipation. In neurasthenia, the muscular tone of the bowels suffers and it becomes incapable of moving the fecal matter onward into the rectum. There are some persons who are persistently constipated without suffering any inconvenience. A patient once told me, in detailing his symptoms, that as far as his bowels were concerned, they were in perfect condition, as they moved regularly once a week. The majority of persons, however, complain that unless they have a daily evacuation they

5

suffer from languor, headache, loss of appetite and depression. So potent an influence does a free evacuation
have on the condition of well-being that even Voltaire
was induced to write: " Those persons who are in good
position . . . whose bowels are freed by an easy, regular, peristaltic movement every morning as soon as they
have breakfasted . . . those who are thus favored by
nature are mild, affable, gracious, kind. A no from
their mouth comes with more grace than a yes from the
mouth of one that is constipated."

A recent German writer has collected a large number of cases of neurasthenia dependent wholly on constipation and the evil results thereof. He contends, and
his contention cannot be questioned, that the bowels
normally manufacture poisons which, when absorbed,
influence the delicate nervous system. Hypochondriacs
are usually constipated, and so are the insane. One
of my patients, who is an habitual sufferer from constipation, and has periodic " nerve storms," finds immediate relief after taking a saline purgative. The physiology of defecation is practically as follows: The fecal
matter formed in the large intestine sets up peristalsis,
which moves the fecal mass through the large bowel,
dropping it into the rectum. At the latter point " a call
of nature " takes place, and evacuation is the result. If
no response is made to this " call " by the individual,
whether through laziness or attention to other duties,
the watery portion of the fecal mass is absorbed, passes
into the circulation and intoxicates the nervous system.
Persons who suffer from this auto-intoxication have a
muddy skin, dark rings under the eyes, cold extremities,
an unpleasant taste in the mouth, dark, offensive and

insufficient bowel movements and a heavy urine, which leaves a deposit on standing.

MUCOUS ENTERITIS is an intestinal neurosis occurring specially in hysteric females and those of a highly neurotic constitution.

The most important symptom associated with severe colicky pain is the passage at varying intervals of long threads of mucus, which are imperfect casts of the gut. The disease is chronic and obstinate to treatment.

SEXUAL SIGNS. When the symptoms of neurasthenia predominate in the sexual apparatus, we speak of sexual neurasthenia. In neurasthenia the sexual power is usually very much diminished, either by incomplete erections, premature ejaculations or night emissions. Married men find this weakness a source of much mental suffering, and the constant fear of impotency prompts them to seek medical advice. It is, without doubt, true that the majority of functional troubles of the sexual organs are of a neurasthenic nature. Whatever the changes may be in his sexual apparatus, the unfortunate sufferer is inclined to exaggerate them by a vivid imagination or the perusal of quack advertisements. Normal ingredients of the urine, such as phosphates and urates, passed by such persons, are declared by charlatans, to be seminal fluid. Although seminal fluid may be passed during urination or defecation, it is nevertheless a rare occurrence.

Involuntary seminal emissions in a healthy unmarried man, occurring at different periods, must always be regarded as an evidence of good health. It is only when the emissions are followed by depression, vague pains in the head, and a feeling of exhaustion, that they are to be regarded as harmful. Some individuals suffer no inconvenience from night emissions, occurring even as often as several times a week, whereas, in others, a simple emission once a week, or even less often, is attended by the signs previously noted. Seminal emissions may be the cause of nerve depression, not the consequence of the loss of semen, but from the nerve exhaustion following. More often, the emissions are the result of nerve depression. It frequently happens that sufferers from seminal emissions attribute their trouble to the habit of self-abuse. While the habit is unfortunately well nigh universal among both sexes and animals, and frequently attended by dire results, the latter have, no doubt, been greatly exaggerated.

Spermatorrhea, or the passing of semen with the urine or during defecation, is indicative of grave debility of the sexual apparatus. It is usually the result of neglected or improperly treated seminal emissions. Many cases of so-called spermatorrhea, it must be emphasized, are really urethral discharges, other than semen. The microscope alone can determine the nature of the discharge.

Impotence signifies one of the following conditions. 1. Deficiency of desire and power. 2. Deficiency of power with increased desire. 3. Abnormal erectile power, known as priapism, in which there is no discharge of semen. Very often the impotence is imaginary, a form known as *psychical impotency*. It is strange that people are not better educated in regard to their sexual functions. All they learn is of a suggestive nature by the reading of erotic literature and quack advertisements. Among the prominent symptoms of sexual neurasthenia, are: dimness of vision, back pains, mental depression and defective memory, dyspepsia, palpitation of the heart and dizziness. In women, sexual neurasthenia presents symptoms similar to those of man, although they occur with less frequency. Some suffer from nocturnal orgasms, accompanied by dreams, and they awake feeling nervous, depressed and exhausted. In married women, the sexual appetite may be increased at first, but it rapidly disappears, to be followed very often by distaste or even disgust.

THE SEXUAL HYPOCHONDRIAC. This unfortunate creature, boy, girl, man or woman, usually lives a life of profound despondency, the result of a real or fancied disturbance of the sexual organs. Such cases demand a true explanation of the disorder, but when the morbid state of mind is encouraged by the charlatan, only dire results follow. There is no sufferer to whom truth is more repellant than the sexual hypochondriac, in fact, his morbid fear is a delusion which he wishes to have verified. The sexual hypochondriac may be the victim of one of the following disorders: Involuntary seminal discharges, impotency, masturbation, or syphilophobia.

Involuntary seminal discharges are quite natural and occur in all persons who lead a correct and continent life, and are not unlike menstruation occurring in women at periodical intervals. The " night emissions " are not necessarily the involuntary discharge of semen, but are often made up of a fluid derived from the prostate gland. Some persons secrete a larger quantity of prostatic fluid than others, hence it is quite within the limits of health for such individuals to have involuntary discharges at more frequent intervals. Then, again, the character of food eaten has a notable influence on the amount of seminal or prostatic fluid secreted. The milky character of the urine in the sexual hypochondriac is not semen but phosphates, a fact which is made evident when a little acid is added to the urine, resulting in the complete disappearance of the milky character of the urine. The mucilage-like fluid observed at the head of the penis, after stool, is often of no consequence, consisting, as it often does, of the secretion of the prostate gland.

Impotency, or fondly called, " lost manhood " by the advertising quack, is in most instances an imaginary condition. True manhood finds no index in the vigor of the sexual apparatus. The more man approaches the condition of brute creation, the more powerful is his sexual instinct.

As man and woman ascend the scale of moral and social life, there is less inclination for the performance of the sexual act. Such individuals are both potent and impotent at times. The best type of a married man is only potent in the presence of his consort. If he demonstrates this potency toward another, his moral standard is as low as the negro who commits rape as often as occasion permits. An indefinite number of unforeseen conditions, like mental and physical fatigue, disgust, worry and anger, conduce to make every man impotent at times. The fear and timidity which possess the newly married are evidences of morality and not sexual weakness. It has been estimated by a trustworthy statistician that at least 60 per cent. of young husbands fail in the first attempt after marriage. There are many individuals who are impotent, owing to their overwhelming fear of contracting some disease. There are persons who manifest impotency toward certain women, but who are fully capable of performing the act with others.

Unnatural practices are bound to be followed by impotency. The sexual act, when aroused by artificial means, finds no response when invoked by natural methods. Sexual psychopathy, or the attainment of sexual desire by unnatural means, is a stigma of degeneration manifested in persons who have inherited or acquired a defective nerve organization, and is common among the insane.

MASTURBATION may conduce to severe disturbances in the mental and physical health, but as the habit is stopped at an early period of life, as soon as the indecency of the habit is explained, no possible consequences ever arise. We must all encounter a period in life when there is a conflict between the passions and one's better self, but the latter is usually the victor in the combat. It is not an exaggeration to maintain, that, in the majority of instances, the evils arising from masturbation practiced moderately, and for a short period in youth, are largely mental, developed from the loss of self-respect and the sense of unmanliness.

FORMS OF NEURASTHENIA. Beard makes the following classification of neurasthenia:

1. Cerebral neurasthenia (cerebrasthenia, cerebral exhaustion).

2. Spinal neurasthenia (myelasthenia, spinal exhaustion).

3. Digestive neurasthenia (nervous dyspepsia).

4. Sexual neurasthenia (sexual exhaustion).

5. Traumatic neurasthenia (traumatic exhaustion).

6. Hemi-neurasthenia (hemi-exhaustion).

7. Hysterical neurasthenia (hysterical exhaustion).

A more modern classification is that of Dana.[20] Here the types of neurasthenia are made dependent upon the age, the sex, and the hereditary endowments of the individual.

PRIMARY NEURASTHENIA. Neurasthenia appearing at the adolescent period is likely to be associated with a primarily weak and nervous constitution. Mental symptoms predominate, assuming the character of hypochondriasis with fixed ideas or morbid fear. Sexual ideas and symptoms likewise predominate.

HYSTERO-NEURASTHENIA. Occurs in women associated with hysteria. Much pain along the back, gives rise to the condition known as " spinal irritation."

ACQUIRED NEURASTHENIA AND LITHEMIA. Here, the element of heredity is less marked, while the extrinsic causes of neurasthenia dominate the situation, viz.: Excessive eating, drinking, shocks, injuries, poisons, syphilis, and gouty tendencies. This form occurs during the active period of life.

CLIMACTERIC. This develops in the middle life and is associated with arterial degeneration and a diminished resistance of the body generally. Physical weakness is greater, associated with vasomotor disturbances, and a tendency to melancholia.

TRAUMATIC NEURASTHENIA. After injuries, however slight, but associated with fright and emotional disturbance, the patient develops all the symptoms of neurasthenia. The latter may consume several weeks in developing, and do not always immediately follow the injury. Such cases usually end in litigation and the worry, incident to the trial, will aggravate the symptoms. After the trial the patient may get well, but this is, by no means, the invariable rule.

SPINAL IRRITATION. In this form, to the picture of neurasthenia is added painful symptoms related chiefly to the sensory nerves of the spine. The pain predominates in the lower part of the back and also in the back of the neck. Exertion intensifies the pain. Relief and comfort seem only to be secured by rest in bed, so they go there and remain.

The spinal processes are sensitive to pressure and the painful points vary at each examination. The arms and legs are exceedingly weak, incapacitating the subject from any kind of exertion.

The duration of the affection may extend into years or their invalidism may become permanent. While the symptoms are essentially referred to the spine, the real trouble has its seat in the brain, which mental sensitiveness aggravates.

NEURASTHENIA WITH FIXED IDEA. This form is associated with a fixed idea of a depressing character relating either to fright or remorse, and worries and harasses the patient through every moment of the waking hours. The fixed idea may center itself on an intense fear of death or that there is an incurable heart or kidney trouble. Such patients may for a time be persuaded to release themselves from their obsession, but it soon recurs, despite all their efforts.

ANGIOPATHIC NEURASTHENIA. Here the vasomotor symptoms predominate. Pulsation or beating of the blood-vessels involves the whole body.

GRAVE NEURASTHENIA. This is characterized by a severe and serious type of exhaustion, both mental and physical. Emaciation is a prominent sign. Only temporary benefit results from treatment, and many of the patients pass into permanent and hopeless invalidism. Men who have reached or passed the middle period of life are the usual subjects, and the condition suggests a premature senescence of the nervous tissues.

DIAGNOSIS. There are several affections closely related to neurasthenia, and the boundary line is very often so severely drawn that a differentiation from them can only be determined by the results of treatment, time, the judgment of the physician, and the willingness of the subject to patiently submit himself as an object of study, of which time is the essence. A better understanding will thus be mutually established between the physician and the patient, for the latter, like all neurasthenics, will agree with Avicenna, " I prefer confidence before art, precepts and all remedies whatever." " Medical art," says Hippocrates, " consists of three things: the patient, his malady, and the physician." Moxon's witty paradox is also apposite. " It is quite as important to know what kind of a patient the disease has got, as to know what sort of a disease the patient has got."

The diagnosis of neurasthenia, or its allied affections, is only warranted after a most painstaking examination of the patient. It is always wise in the examination of the subjects to regard neurasthenia merely as a symptom rather than a disease, and to seek for some local disturbance which reflexly instigates the nervous symptoms. This statement may not receive the sanction of conventionalism, but evidence is rapidly accumulating in support of this contention. The following affections suggest differentiation: 1. Hysteria, 2. Hypochondriasis. 3. Melancholia. 4. General paresis. 5. Insanity.

No physician can afford to depend on any single method in diagnosis. Pathognomonic signs are as uncommon as specific drugs in disease, and the truly skilled diagnostician is he who is catholic and eclectic in the selection of his methods, and the most painstaking in their application.

THE PATHOGNOMONIC SYMPTOMS OF THE VARIOUS AFFECTIONS.

NEURASTHENIA. Fatigue is the primary and fundamental symptom, relieved by rest and intensified by exertion. There is always a cause, notably over use and abuse of functional activity abetted by a nervous system, which responds readily to irritants, but does not recover in like ratio. The perverse reaction of the irritable, weakened nerve apparatus is characterized by sensory, motor, vasomotor and psychic disturbances. The prognosis is favorable.

HYSTERIA. Neurasthenia in men is in many respects the equivalent of hysteria in women, modified by sex, and with symptoms less developed. In hysteria there is diminished control over the emotions, and the symptoms occur in paroxysms (*nerve storms*) although in the inter-paroxysmal period, the stigmata of the affection are nearly always evident, viz: hysterogenic zones, areas of anesthesia, hyperesthesia, etc. There is a tendency to practice deception, a morbid craving for sympathy, and a perversion of the moral nature. The affection is of indefinite duration, although the hysterical temperament lasts a lifetime.

HYPOCHONDRIASIS. Confined almost exclusively to the male. An isolated mental disturbance with a groundless fear of disease, which has no real existence, but exists only in the imagination of the patient. Hypochondriacs are bodily well with few or no stigmata of neurasthenia. The cause is usually a solitary or sedentary life. There is an hereditary taint. It begins gradually and runs an even course of indefinite duration. The patient does not relax in his endeavors to seek a remedy for his imaginary affection.

MELANCHOLIA. In the early stages of this affection there is a close resemblance to neurasthenia, and the latter has been frequently defined as an abortive form of melancholia. The rapid emaciation, frequent pulse, persistent insomnia, extreme mental depression with delusions and suicidal tendencies are signs which distinguish this affection from neurasthenia.

GENERAL PARESIS. The symptoms of neurasthenia in the primary stage are often responsible for errors in diagnosis. In paresis, however, the mental disturbances are more pronounced. Failure of memory, with expansiveness of ideas, inability to write and spell correctly, tremor of the face, hands and tongue, and unequal pupils are signs which suggest paresis.

Folsom's diagnostic description of the early stages of paresis is worthy of citation: " It should arouse suspicion if, for instance, a strong, healthy man, in or near the prime of life, distinctly not of the nervous, neurotic or neurasthenic type, shows some loss of interest in his affairs or impaired faculty of attending to them; if he becomes varyingly absent-minded, heedless, indifferent, negligent, apathetic, inconsiderate, and although able to follow his routine duties, his ability to take up new work is, no matter how little, diminished; if he can less well command mental attention and concentration, conception, perception, reflection, judgment; if there is an unwonted lack of initiative, and if exertion causes unwonted mental and physical fatigue; if the emotions are intensified and easily change, or are excited readily from trifling causes; if the sexual instinct is not reasonably controlled; if the finer feelings are even slightly blunted; if the person in question regards with placid apathy his own acts of indifference and irritability and their consequences, and especially if at times he sees himself in his true light, and suddenly fails again to do so; if any symptoms of cerebral vasomotor disturbances are noticed, however vague or variable."

INSANITY. Savill,[21] in his excellent treatise, refers to a mental disorder which is special to neurasthenia. The recognition of such a mental state is of the utmost importance, as such patients require no restraint nor asylum treatment. It differs from true insanity in six respects:

1. Marked bodily weakness precedes and accompanies the disorder.

2. The condition is curable by appropriate measures after a duration of a few weeks or months.

3. The most prominent feature of the mental condition is mental weakness. Delusions and hallucinations, as a rule, are absent.

4. It is difficult to make it correspond with any of the types of insanity found in asylums.

5. The mental symptoms vary from day to day, and lucid intervals occur from time to time, during which a casual observer might find nothing wrong with them.

6. There is no family history of insanity.

PROGNOSIS. As a rule, neurasthenia is a curable disease. The duration and permanency of cure is a matter based on the individual treated and the judgment of the physician in the application of his resources. The individual must be regarded from the following standpoints:

1. History of heredity.

2. His nerve capital.
3. His environment.
4. His habits.

First of all, *heredity* plays only a subordinate rôle in neurasthenia, provided the patient can be made conscious of the fact, that nerve health is a matter of individual effort in the direction of rigid regard of hygienic laws. If there is an abundance of reserve *nerve capital,* a few weeks or months, will suffice to restore the individual to a condition of well-being. *Environment* and *habits* determine the permanency of a cure and relapses. If the patient subjects himself after recovery to the causes which induced his disease, he soon suffers from another attack of nervous breakdown, drifts into a state of chronic invalidism or becomes an habitue of some drug habit.   An attack of neurasthenia cripples a nervous system, and predisposes to other attacks, so that eternal vigilance becomes the keynote of health.   As a rule, however, the neurasthenic enjoys a long life, for he is ever conscious of his past experience, which guides him safely along the pathway of hygienic living.   Of consumption, one has truly said, `` If I knew what produced it, I could cure it.''   Just so with neurasthenia, we know what will produce it, but do we give due regard to the details in the patient's life history, any one of which, if not eliminated, will suffice to perpetuate the disease ?   Our standard of progress is not evidenced by the introduction of new drugs, the delirium of which threatens to annihilate rational therapeutics.   Reliance on the healing power of nature is an evidence of erudition.   It affords the discerning physician an opportunity of knowing what not to do, and enables him to apply the highest principles of the therapeutic art.

SUMMARY.

1. Fatigue and the proneness to it is the primary and essential sign of neurasthenia. It is relieved by rest and instigated by exertion.

2. Neurasthenia is a functional disease, and the exclusion of organic disease is absolutely essential before the diagnosis of neurasthenia is warranted. Disease is the sphinx of medicine. The interpretation of the signs constitutes diagnosis, which is the Œdipus of medicine. The translation may be correct, partially correct or wrong. In all three instances, the result, as far as the patient is concerned, will, as a rule, be the same, provided no treatment is instituted. To treat a disease, other than by expectant methods, where the diagnosis is in question, is adding insult to injury.

3. The objective are subsidiary to the subjective symptoms in neurasthenia, for it is more often necessary to know " what kind of a patient the disease has got, as to know what sort of a disease the patient has got."

4. The patient who expects the physician to make an immediate diagnosis, is a believer in miracles and, carrying his absurdity to extremes, predicts like results from treatment. Such a patient should be admonished to consult Providence and not a physician, for he is as mad as his nerves.

5. Neurasthenia lies on the borderland of insanity, and if the patient is not even mildly insane, his symptoms are often severe enough to make him so.

6. The prognosis is dependent on a multitude of factors: the patient, his habits, the cause of his disease, the severity of reaction on the part of his nervous system, etc. As a rule, the prognosis is good, for the logical

tendency of a pathologic condition is always toward a physiologic ending.

"But, after all, I am a man, and not a theorem. A system cannot suffer, but I suffer. Logic makes only one demand—that of consequence; but life makes a thousand; the body wants health, the imagination cries out for beauty, and the heart for love; pride asks for consideration, the soul yearns for peace, the conscience for holiness; our whole being is athirst for happiness and for perfection; and we, tottering, mutilated, and incomplete, cannot always feign philosophic insensibility; we stretch out our arms toward life, and we say to it under our breath, ' Why—why—hast thou deceived me ? ' "—HENRI FREDERIC AMIEL.

And, I may append to the foregoing, because thou hast deceived nature.

CHAPTER V.

THE GENERAL TREATMENT OF NEURASTHENIA.

OBJECTS OF TREATMENT.—ELIMINATION OF FACTORS
CONDUCIVE TO THE DISEASE.—TREATMENT OF THE
DISEASE. — CLIMATE. — TREATMENT OF THE SYMP-
TOMS: INSOMNIA, HEART, STOMACH, INTESTINAL, AND
SEXUAL SYMPTOMS.—HYPNOTISM AS A MODE OF CURE.

THE physiologic treatment of neurasthenia in general
aims to fulfil the following objects: 1. The removal of
the cause; 2. The treatment of the disease; 3. The
treatment of symptoms.

Under physiologic treatment is comprised the use of
remedial measures, other than the use of drugs, by
which the natural powers of the human body are so-
licited to combat disease. These natural measures cannot be supplanted by the most skilful drugging, and
should be employed by the progressive physician to the
exclusion of drugs in such a disease as neurasthenia.
The monumental work of Solomon Solis Cohen, entitled
" A System of Physiologic Therapeutics," recently issued in eleven octavo volumes, is an enduring tribute
to the value of physiologic therapeutics.

ELIMINATION OF FACTORS CONDUCIVE TO NEURAS-
THENIA. The ideal aim of the physician is unquestionably the removal of the cause of neurasthenia, but even

though this is possible, there yet remains the disease, the effect of the cause, which must claim attention.

Sleep is, without doubt, the natural restorative of a fagged brain. The writer, when suffering from brain tire, finds more relief by three day's absolute rest in bed than by a sojourn of two weeks in the country after the conventional manner. Sleep is, however, a restorative that cannot always be summoned at will. The inventor, speculator, student and business man must seek mental recreation. The brain worker who seeks diversion and does so constrainedly defeats the object of such diversion. The diversion adopted must be agreeable. Travel is often suggested as a method of mental recreation, but it is often done in such a perfunctory way that the victim returns to his habitual routine work more exhausted than recuperated. "They may change their skies, but not themselves." Indulgence in extraneous literature, the cultivation of a fad, some regulated exercise, like golf, bicycling, hunting, etc., are excellent means of diversion. Employment prevents melancholy—it is restful to the body. Inaction, idleness and the constant pursuit of pleasure, simply encourage premature old age. Above all things in seeking physical exercises as a means of diversion, one must be sure to avoid physical overwork. Physical exhaustion is naught else but nervous fatigue, for every physical act is the result of nervous energy. The limit of physical exercise is fatigue. Rational exercise is not nerve exertion, but a gradual and progressive use of muscles, diverting the blood from the overtaxed brain throughout the entire body. Neurasthenics, who over-exercise, develop poisons equally as injurious as those generated by brain strain.

RELIEF FOR WORRIMENT. " Worry, not work, kills." Worry in persons previously unaccustomed to great responsibilities is one of the greatest factors in the premature loss of health and life. Worry, grief, passion and fretting are powerful nervous shocks. They arrest the functions of digestion and impair the bodily functions.

SELF-CONTROL is a resourceful palladium against nervous prostration. The latter affection is rarely encountered in those who have acquired a knowledge of self-government. I refer to neurasthenia, incited by worry, fretting, and emotional disturbances of any kind. From what has preceded, we already know that there are forms of neurasthenia which develop and are beyond the control of the individual. Man has been defined as " a creature looking before and after." He must know what his powers and limitations are before he can intelligently exercise them to the benefit of his mind and body. Man, by his unbridled indulgence of his passions, is continually paying the penalty for his sacrifice of self-control. We must, therefore, guard ourselves from drifting upon the shoals of nervous degradation. When nervous breakdown once occurs, recovery is only possible to a certain extent, and relapses are frequent. As Courtney put it: " Hardly any of them come out of the conflict unscathed, and though many recover sufficiently to cope with the ordinary duties and trials of life, they are never quite capable of weathering its real storms."

THE TREATMENT OF THE DISEASE.

THE REST CURE. In a little book, " Fat and Blood and How to Make Them," Dr. Weir Mitchell has created a new era in curative medicine, and the victims of nervous prostration and hysteria are his debtors. He has simplified a task heretofore almost impossible of attainment, viz.: The cure of a pronounced case of nervous prostration. It would be ridiculous to affirm that all cases can be cured by the rest cure, any more than to say that any method of treatment, yet devised, will cure all cases of the disease to which it is adapted. This much one can conscientiously and conservatively say—it cures and benefits a large percentage of cases where the dominant causative factor is overwork, resulting from a perennial unrest of body and mind, while in a small percentage of cases, it aggravates rather than benefits the disease. For instance, in splanchnic neurasthenia, as well as in other forms, the rest cure alone, gives only temporary relief, insomuch as the therapeutic manœuvres incident to the rest cure increase the resistance of the nervous system, and make it less responsive to a multitude of irritants.

The cardinal points of the rest cure are isolation of the patient, rest with exercise and over-feeding. A rest cure attempted at the patient's home is rarely attended with success, hence the necessity of absolute isolation, that is, the execution of the cure away from home to obtain the necessary control of the patient. The most important element of treatment is moral control. Loving and sympathetic relatives can never appreciate the nature of the patient's symptoms. There are some patients who thrive poorly on absolute isolation, in which instances they are occasionally permitted to see at intervals their friends and members of their family. An intelligent nurse is indispensable—a poor nurse is worse than useless. The details of the method are essentially as follows: The patient is confined to bed, and under no circumstances is allowed to get up, to read, or write. The patient is even fed by the nurse, the object being to secure perfect passivity of mind and body. Absolute rest is not always enforced, the method being modified to suit the individual case. It is the rule for patients to affirm that it is impossible for them to remain in bed continuously, and it is but natural that they should make this statement, for their extreme restlessness only announces the instability of their nervous system. Contrary evidence is soon forthcoming after absolute rest in bed and the manifestations of nerve irritability are subdued. It is then that they share the enthusiasm of the poet, when they proclaim: "O, bed! O, bed! delicious bed! That heaven upon earth to the weary head!"

After rest in bed for several weeks the patient is allowed to sit up. To facilitate digestion and build up nutrition during the rest cure, massage and electricity are employed daily. Massage and electricity give exercise to the unused muscles, improve the circulation and promote the absorption of nourishment. Insomuch, as nearly all neurasthenics suffer from indigestion, and consequently imperfect body nourishment, diet is a most important factor in the rest treatment. Great discretion must be exercised by the physician in the selection of the proper diet, and when this is accomplished, it is surprising what prodigious quantities of food can be taken by the patient undergoing the rest cure. The improvement in nutrition is manifested by increase in weight, which may be all the way from 10 to 40 pounds. In many individuals hydropathic treatment is employed, with water at varying degrees of temperature, and it is surprising to note the sedative and tonic influences of cold water when the patient is accustomed to its use.

(THE PARTIAL REST TREATMENT.) In cases of mild neurasthenia, and for patients who cannot give up their entire time to the full rest treatment, which is often the case in men, the following partial rest treatment may be employed: On waking in the morning, a cup of cocoa is taken, and the patient should remain in bed twenty minutes longer; after this, the patient rises and takes a cool or cold sponge or shower bath, after which the skin is vigorously rubbed with a rough towel; following the bath, breakfast is taken, after which the patient should lie down for an hour and remain at absolute rest, without reading. At 10:30, a glass of milk is taken, when the patient may go out for a walk or drive or attend to business. At 1 o'clock luncheon or dinner is taken, after which meal the patient should lie down for an hour. In the afternoon any recreation may be taken, or attention paid to business until 6:30, when dinner or supper is taken, followed by rest for an hour. At 9:30 the patient should retire for the night. Massage should be taken once a day; before rising in the morning, after the morning cup of cocoa, or in the evening before retiring. A wineglassful of malt should be taken with each meal, and if the patient has impoverished blood, some simple iron preparation should be taken. In conclusion, "It is reiterated," says Courtney, "that affections of the brain and nervous system are in greater measure preventable than those of other parts; consequently the mental and nervous salvation of the individual is, practically speaking, to a very marked extent, within his own hands, and may be worked out by him through rigid attention to the guidance of hygienic laws."

THE TREATMENT OF SYMPTOMS.—INSOMNIA.

THE THEORIES OF SLEEP. The *anemic theory* supposes that during sleep there is a decreased amount of blood in the brain. The *toxic theory* supposes that in consequence of the wear and tear of the body tissues, waste products are generated which have a benumbing influence on the brain cells, which preside over the senses. A strong proof of the latter hypothesis is adduced by the following observation of Strümpell: A young man had lost all power of sensation except in the right eye and the left ear. When the former was covered by a bandage and the latter stopped by a plug the brain of the subject was practically isolated from the outer world, and the invariable result was genuine sleep. "The substance of the brain," says Hammond, in "Sleep and Its Derangements," "is consumed by every thought, by every action of the will, by every sound that is heard, by every object that is seen, by every odor that is smelled, by every painful or pleasurable sensation, and soon each instance of our lives witnesses the decay of some portion of its mass and the formation of new material to take its place."

During sleep the physical and mental functions are at rest. Sleep is more essential to life than food. In sleep, muscular relaxation is absolute, and the amount of air inspired by a normal man is one-seventh of that used during similar periods of quiet wakefulness. The pulse is less rapid, and the brain contains less blood. The first few hours of sleep are the most valuable, because they are most profound.

AMOUNT OF SLEEP NECESSARY. In the time of Solomon, the twenty-four hours were divided into three parts—eight hours for labor and occupation, eight hours for rest, refreshment and recreation and surcease of all labor, and eight hours for sleep. The object of sleep is the reconstruction of overworked organs, and it would be too arbitrary to determine the number of hours necessary for sleep, for its real value lies more in the intensity of sleep than on its duration. Again, the amount of sleep necessary is commensurate with the mental and physical exercise of the waking hours. Eight hours of a disturbed, dreamy sleep is barely the equivalent of two hours of a deep, dreamless sleep. For this reason, we can easily understand why men of the greatest mental activity are usually the briefest sleepers. Frederick the Great required only five hours' sleep, and Pitt only three hours. Brown says, that at four years, twelve hours' sleep are needed; at fourteen years, ten hours; at seventeen, nine and one-half hours; then seven or eight hours during adult life. In old age, continuous sleep is rare and the necessity less; but frequent naps during the day and night make up the average. In cold countries more sleep is required than in warm climates. The length of time a person can live without sleep is about three weeks.

CONDITIONS FAVORING SLEEP. A well ventilated room, cool, dark and quiet. A comfortable bed with a moderate amount of covering. Mental worries and intense thoughts interfere with sleep. Sleep is a powerful habit. A person who awakens at a certain hour for several successive nights, eventually establishes the habit of awakening at that hour. The habit should be cultivated of retiring and awakening at a definite hour.

THE CAUSE OF INSOMNIA OR SLEEPLESSNESS. Prof. See divides all causes of insomnia into: 1. Psychical, and 2. Physical. The causes of psychical insomnia include cases of sleeplessness dependent on mental emotion, to thought, worry, that is, to causes not directly dependent on organic disease. Young, the well-known author of " Night Thoughts," was presumably thus afflicted—

" From short as usual and disturbed repose,
I awake. How happy those that wake no more ;
I awake emerging from a sea of dreams
Tumultuous, where my wrecked despondent thought
From wave to wave of fancied misery
At random drove, her helm of reason lost ! "

The worries of the student, the merchant, the speculator, homesickness and disappointments are of this order. In the treatment of such cases, the physician is often powerless to act.

" Who shall minister to a mind diseased ;
Pluck from the memory a rooted sorrow,
'Rase out the written troubles of the brain,
And with some sweet oblivious antidote
Cleanse the stuffed bosom of that perilous stuff
Which weighs upon the heart ? "

PHYSICAL CAUSES. Every deviation of health is characterized by disturbance of sleep, but in most cases where a vicious sleep habit is established, it tends to persist. Among the chief causes are: 1. Brain strain; 2. Organic diseases of the brain and arteries; 3. Stomach and intestinal diseases; 4. Irritation of the sexual organs; 5. Poisonous substances (toxic insomnia).

THE INSOMNIA OF BRAIN STRAIN. This means increase in the supply of blood to the brain, eventuating in cerebral congestion. It is an undoubted fact, that the brain strain of severe mental labor is measurably lessened by an adequate amount of physical exercises. Physiologists and hygienists have shown this to be true, yet we must be cautious in going to the other extreme, taking too much physical exercise; for otherwise, the poisonous substances generated by muscular fatigue only tend to excite the brain and tend to insomnia.

THE INSOMNIA OF ORGANIC DISEASES OF THE BRAIN AND ARTERIES. Whenever the nutrition of the brain is compromised by actual disease, then insomnia of an aggravating and persistent character results. When the insomnia is caused by brain congestion, there is flushing of the face, redness of the eyes, giddiness, confusion of ideas, and sometimes stupor. Insanity may commence with obstinate insomnia.

THE INSOMNIA OF STOMACH AND INTESTINAL DISEASE. In indigestion, toxic substances are developed which irritate the brain and prevent sleep. In many instances, the accumulation of gases in the stomach and intestines by pressing on important organs, notably the heart and lungs, induce sleeplessness indirectly. Some persons sleep best, if, before retiring, they take a light repast; others, on the contrary, would find such a procedure an indiscretion, certain to be followed by insomnia. Sleep after eating is a salutary procedure. It draws the blood from the brain to the stomach, and thus facilitates digestion.

TOXIC INSOMNIA. Insomnia induced by the indiscriminate use of poisonous substances like alcohol, coffee, tea, tobacco, etc. Not infrequently the inhibition of any one of these substances will often cure an intractable insomnia.

SYMPTOMS OF INSOMNIA. In the insomnia of neurasthenia, the sleep is often interrupted by dreams of the most abhorrent nature, which seem to dominate the person in the wakeful state. As a result of insomnia, many neurasthenics are restless, excited, querulous and irritable.

TREATMENT OF INSOMNIA. It has been truly said that if sleep and hope should be taken from man, he would be the most miserable being in existence. Much can be obtained by obeying the laws of hygiene. Attention must be directed to a minute investigation of all the bodily functions to ascertain the fundamental condition, of which insomnia is a mere manifestation. We possess many drugs which, when prescribed with discretion, may be regarded as harmless, yet drugs should only be used as a last resort, for any drug which induces sleep by overpowering the body is not entirely without danger.

The bromides are the safest hypnotics, and so are, lupulin, valerian and spirits of lavender. The use of other hypnotics is fraught with danger, and should never be prescribed until one has exhausted every other simpler means to produce sleep, for of all beings the neurasthenic is specially liable to succumb to a drug habit.

Generally speaking, an adequate amount of physical exercise is necessary in all sufferers from insomnia. Nothing is more conducive to sleep than exercise taken in the open air. Some diversion for the brain worker may be found in change of scene and society. " Seeing that too much sadness has congealed your blood, and melancholy is the nurse of frenzy, therefore, have thought it good for you to hear a play, and frame your mind to mirth and merriment, which bars a thousand harms and lengthens life."

No detail should be neglected in ascertaining the cause of insomnia. Tea or coffee should not be taken at the evening meal, and tobacco should not be used, at least some hours before retiring. A glass of warm milk, or a cup of hot bouillon before retiring may prove beneficial in inducing sleep. Some derive sleep by taking a glass of beer or malt extract before retiring. If the sufferer from insomnia be a literary man or student, all intellectual effort should be stopped at least an hour before retiring, and the interval filled in with some extraneous dull reading. When this fails, no intellectual work should be done after supper, reserving that work for the early morning hours. Some cases of insomnia only yield after a complete change of scene free from excitement and sightseeing. Active exercise before retiring, with dumb-bells, pulley-weights or Indian clubs, followed by a tepid or warm sponge bath, often induces healthful and refreshing sleep. Climate is an essential consideration in those who suffer from insomnia. Warm climates are soothing, and cool climates stimulating to the nervous system. On account of the cool nights in the mountainous districts, refreshing sleep can often be obtained. Some find benefit by residing at the seashore. California has a marvelous diversity of surface and corresponding varieties of climate. While the climate of southern California is especially favorable for consumptives or persons with heart or kidney diseases, northern California is better adapted to build up the neurasthenic. The winds that sweep through the Golden Gate often make the summer climate of San Francisco somewhat harsh, yet there are districts in the immediate vicinity of San Francisco free from winds and fogs, and there is no city in the world which has such environs. About 125 miles from San Francisco, at Monterey, is the famous Del Monte hotel. Here the climate is sedative and equable, and permits of an out-door life throughout the year. The temperature rarely rises above 80° F. The temperature of the water averages 52° F. in January and 60° F. in July. Neurasthenics, who suffer from insomnia, obtain much relief at Monterey, where art has conspired with Nature to make this one of the garden-spots of the world.

HYDROTHERAPY is a valuable adjunct in the treatment of insomnia. Schneller's experiments proved conclusively that ice applied to the head of an animal caused contraction of the blood vessels of the brain, which persisted for a short time after the ice was removed. The brief application of cold or warm water to the surface of the body is stimulating, but if prolonged, depressant. A cool sponge bath, or even a cold plunge before retiring, will provoke sleep. The secondary effect of cold to the skin, is to dilate the blood-vessels, which draws the blood away from the brain. Many sufferers find relief in a prolonged warm bath before retiring, the effect being sedative on the nervous system. Others find equal benefit in a hot foot bath. Some find relief in a Turkish bath, followed by a general massage. The wet pack has done heroic service for many nervous persons. It is used as follows: A sheet having been wrung out of cold water, is thrown over the patient from neck to ankles, and over this several dry blankets, with a hot-water bag to the feet and a cold wet cloth to the forehead. The patient remains in the pack from half an hour to an hour, and is then vigorously rubbed with a coarse, dry cloth until the skin glows. The wet pack may be given every night or several times a week.

Hot compresses, consisting of flannels wrung out of hot water, applied to the abdomen and covered with dry flannels, are often efficacious. A hot bag may be substituted. The cold douche to the head, or a shower bath to the head and spine, are frequently serviceable.

MASSAGE is often of service in insomnia, when every other hygienic measure fails.

Some persons can induce sleep by having recourse to the hop pillow, which should be moistened with spirits before being placed under the head of the patient. Among drugs, bromide of potash is the least harmful. For an adult, 30 grains may be taken in sweetened water before retiring, and repeated in an hour, if necessary. It is especially useful in nervous cases.

ELECTRICITY, when properly employed, especially in the form of static electricity, is almost an indispensable remedy in insomnia. Contrary results often follow its injudicious application. The Galvanic current has a tendency to make some persons sleepy, and is to be applied in the evening. The Faradic current makes most people wakeful. Electricity is especially useful in insomnia of brain strain and alcoholism.

HYPNOTISM is likewise an indispensable agent when judiciously employed.

A common procedure for inducing sleep is energetic and frequently repeated opening and closing of the eyelids. Auto-suggestion is often of service. The patient should go to bed with the firm conviction that sleep is bound to follow. One may imagine observing all the phenomena incident to sleep in another person. The reading of dull books or concentrating the mind on some blank and wearying picture makes the mind receptive to only one suggestion, viz, sleep.

> " A flock of sheep that leisurely pass by
> One after one ; the sound of rain and bees
> Murmuring ; the fall of rivers, winds and seas,
> Smooth fields, white sheets of water and pure skies."

DREAMS. These are frequent concomitants of the neurasthenic state. Dreams are not recalled when sleep is profound, but occurring at the natural time of waking they are remembered. Dreams are made up of ideas and emotions, which have no laws of association nor coherence. In ancient times, dreams were regarded with much significance, but the attempts of the scientist to classify them has been attended with indifferent results. Diseases of the liver are supposed to be associated with dreams of disturbed forms.

NIGHTMARE. This may prove indicative of an irritation somewhere in the organism, especially so in nervous individuals. Sleeping on the back induces it. The causes of nightmare embrace almost all bodily ailments, notably digestive disturbances, heart disease, worry and excitement.

TREATMENT OF THE HEART SYMPTOMS.

PALPITATION OF THE HEART. Absolute rest in bed in a large ventilated and darkened chamber with the clothing removed. The application of an ice-bag to the region of the heart or cloths saturated in cold water are very effective agents. Swallowing small pieces of ice or drinking large draughts of cold water or a glass of hot water, are procedures frequently adopted. To prevent attacks of palpitation, excitement of all kinds must be avoided, and tea, coffee, and alcohol must be discontinued or at least reduced. When the palpitation is dependent on impoverished blood, iron in some form is serviceable. When a stomach disturbance is at the bottom of the trouble, it must be cured. Electricity is an effective agent. It should be given, if possible, twice a day in the form of Galvanism; the positive pole on the back of the neck and the negative drawn along the course of the pneumogastric nerves in the neck. Some cases are benefited by residence at high altitudes, others, by a sea voyage. Not infrequently the application of cold to the spine will arrest a paroxysm. When everything else fails, the rest cure often yields good results.

TREATMENT OF THE STOMACH AND INTESTINAL SYMPTOMS.

NERVOUS DYSPEPSIA. In the majority of instances, indigestion is caused by too rapid eating and the consumption of too much food. Digestion begins in the mouth. This is especially true of the digestion of starchy foods. Many dyspeptics are cured of their evil by thoroughly masticating their food. A meal should be regarded as a pastime, not a necessity, It is difficult and even impossible to lay down any definite rule for the kind of food to be consumed, for "one man's food is another man's poison." The nervous dyspeptic is, as a rule, poorly nourished. It is absurd to suppose that nervous prostration can be cured without increasing and making the nourishment effective. This statement refers to the qualitative and not the quantitative consumption of food. An exhausted nervous system demands a plentiful supply of good nutritious food. Beard maintains, in his classic work on " Sexual neurasthenia," that flesh is the natural food of man. His theory of diet is founded on the theory of evolution, and finds expression in the following three propositions: 1. Living beings feed on that which is below them in the scale of development; 2. The best food for man is that which is just below him or nearest to him in the scale of development; 3. Food is difficult of assimilation for man in proportion to its distance below him in the scale of development. It is undoubtedly true, that those who subsist exclusively upon meat are capable of greater mental and physical exertion than those who consume vegetable food. Animal food contains the greatest variety of nutriment and is generally most easily digested. Beef is more nutritious and stimulating than mutton. The flesh of very young animals is less nutritious, and more difficult of digestion than the flesh of the matured animal. Oysters are very nutritious and digestible when consumed raw. Oatmeal is a frequent cause of indigestion in the nervous dyspeptic. Eggs, milk and fish are very nutritious. When the dyspepsia is severe, an exclusive milk diet for several weeks proves curative. The daily amount necessary must never be less than three pints, and as much as a gallon. A large glassful should be drunk slowly every hour, and, when toleration is established, this amount may be increased at shorter intervals. The digestibility of the milk may be increased by adding a pinch of salt or a teaspoonful of lime water to each glass. Some prefer taking the milk diluted with water or seltzer. When whole milk is loathsome, it may be skimmed or substituted by buttermilk or koumys. Farinaceous foods should, as a rule, be excluded, as they create flatulency and heartburn. Too much liquid should not be taken at

7

a meal, as it dilutes the gastric juice and inhibits digestion. Hygienic measures, such as exercise and bathing, are indispensable, for, by increasing the tone of the nervous system, they indirectly improve digestion. Sufferers from nervous dyspepsia will find material aid by carrying out the partial rest treatment, and confining themselves to the following diet, which excludes starchy foods, which are notoriously indigestible in neurasthenic persons.

On waking, eight ounces of equal parts of hot milk and seltzer water, taken slowly. Breakfast, steak or loin chops with fat, soft-boiled or poached egg, cream toast (very little), half a pint of milk and a small cup of coffee. Lunch, 10 A. M., small teacup of squeezed beef juice with stale bread. 12M., rest or sleep. Midday meal, 12 : 30 P. M., fish, chicken, scraped meat ball, stale bread with plenty of butter, baked apples and cream, two glasses of milk. Lunch, 4 P. M., bottle of koumys, raw scraped beef sandwich or goblet of milk. 5 : 30 P. M., meat or fresh soup, roast or mutton, game, stale bread (sparingly), fresh vegetables (excepting potatoes). Eat slowly, chew the food thoroughly, and never eat when excited or exhausted. Poorly prepared meals are often a source of dyspepsia. Washing the stomach by means of a tube is often indicated for the relief of dyspepsia. Constipation is frequently a cause of dyspepsia and loss of appetite.

Personally, I have observed only temporary good to result from the use of such agents as pepsin, pancreatin and hydrochloric acid. To stimulate digestion, strychnin is often invaluable. The addition of common salt to our food stimulates digestion. Alcohol should be stopped, although there can be no objection to a moderate use of some light wine taken with meals.

RULES FOR DYSPEPTICS.

RULE I. Eat slowly and chew the food thoroughly. If the foregoing are not observed, then the rule of Sir Andrew Clark should be followed, viz.: Count the bites. For every mouthful of meat thirty-two bites must be allowed, or one bite to every tooth. If the meat is tough, sixty-four bites must be allowed, and ninety-six bites, if very tough. This rule is an almost positive protection against dyspepsia, dependent on hurried eating, and will, in most instances, cure the disease.

RULE II. Solids and liquids must be taken at separate times. Liquid taken with food in those with weak stomachs dilutes the gastric juice and retards digestion. Then again, when liquids are not taken with the food it induces the patient to chew the food thoroughly, or otherwise it cannot be swallowed. If at breakfast, tea or coffee must be drunk, it is better taken at the completion of the meal.

RULE III. Farinaceous and proteid foods should not be taken at the same meal, in other words, the same character of food only should be introduced into the stomach at the same meal. For example: Bread and butter may be taken at breakfast, but no meat, fish or eggs. Luncheon should consist of fish, eggs or meat, but no bread, potatoes or other farinaceous food. Supper should consist of the same kind of food as at luncheon, or farinaceous food only. Introducing the same kind of food into the stomach at each meal insures the completion of digestion at the same time, and not at different times, as would be the case, if the character of the food taken at a meal is different.

Rule iv. If liquid must be taken at a meal, the best drink is hot water, taken on rising in the morning, at 12 o'clock, and again at 4 p. m. Taken at these intervals, there will be no dilution of the gastric juice, and the contents of the previous meal will be washed out of the stomach.

Treatment of Constipation. Each case of constipation must be investigated as an individual one. Habit is an important factor. The desire to go to stool must never be neglected, in fact, it is to be encouraged by a systematic habit of going to the toilet every morning, whether or not the desire is present. Such a practice will often cure the costive habit. Many persons find that a cigar or a pipe after breakfast acts as a laxative. Massage of the abdomen is constantly practiced, but I confess never to have seen any good results from its use, save in children and very young persons. Many persons succeed in obtaining a daily evacuation by taking certain articles of food. Fruit, raw or cooked, taken at breakfast, is often effectual. Some find oatmeal or brown bread to have a similar effect.

It is necessary for the patient to secure bowel action to have in the intestines a certain bulk of fecal matter. The sparing use of vegetables, fruits and water will produce a small residue of undigested matter, hence it is necessary to partake of food which contains a large amount of cellulose, which remaining undigested, fills the bowels and provokes vigorous peristalsis. Such food consists of vegetables, fruits, coarse breads and water. The vegetables that possess laxative properties, are: spinach, lettuce, tomatoes, Spanish onions and cabbage. Honey and molasses, taken alone or with other food, are frequently laxative. Some people find that coffee is likewise laxative. Fruit, as a laxative, is most efficient when eaten alone, either before retiring or an hour before breakfast. Sweet cider is loosening to the bowels, whereas tea often constipates. Water should be drunk in abundance, especially before retiring or on rising in the morning. Others find that a glass of raw milk taken before breakfast will act as a laxative. Exercise is of great value, especially exercise like horseback riding, which brings the abdominal muscles into play. The continued use of purgatives is a dangerous practice. They are only temporary in action, and make the bowels more constipated than ever. The least objectionable agents of this class are the natural purgative waters, like Carlsbad and Hunyadi Janos. In California we possess an effective natural water called Bythinia. Suppositories of glycerin or a daily enema of cold water is of great value. The same may be said of olive oil. Glycerin (a tablespoonful to four tablespoonfuls), thrown into the rectum is very effective. Cold sponging and baths are valuable additions to the measures suggested.

TREATMENT OF SEXUAL NEURASTHENIA.

CONJUGAL HYGIENE. Normal sexual intercourse is the most powerful passion of human nature, conducive to strong and vigorous health. When followed by a feeling of well-being, it is healthful, but, if, on the contrary, it is followed by depression, the act is harmful. Unnatural methods of intercourse, such as withdrawal, use of condoms and prolongation of the act, are especially harmful, and are often the essential cause of a protracted siege of sexual neurasthenia. It must not be forgotten that the health of the offspring is largely de-

pendent on the condition of the parents at the time of
the conception, and for this reason, the laws of sexual
hygiene should be observed most rigorously. Spitzka
affirms that "children begotten by a drunken father
have repeatedly been found to be epileptic, imbecile,
deaf, mute or insane." Undue repetition of the sexual
act is repugnant to the moral sense, and is certain to
be followed by evil consequences. Sexual intercourse
is intended for the purpose of reproduction, and the
prevention of conception is an injustice to society and
results in injury to both sexes.

The treatment of seminal emissions is generally a
simple matter, when conducted by the physician. Aside
from local measures, the building up of the nervous system is an absolute essential. To arrest the emissions
entirely in a continent unmarried man is an impossi-
bility. What can be really achieved is this, to allow
the emissions to continue without any detriment to
health. Marriage, while offering immunity in the majority of instances, is not invariably productive of such
results, for there are many married men who continue
to have emissions. This is, of course, usually unnatural,
and often indicates that the strength of the organs is
imperfect, or because no real pleasure is derived from
the act, or because there still remain traces of former
sexual troubles. Before emissions can be controlled,
sexual excitement and masturbation must be avoided.
The diet should be non-stimulating. Spices, alcoholic
drinks, strong coffee and tea must not be used. Before
retiring, very little fluid or food should be taken. Sleep
should not be prolonged, and early rising is important.
The patient should never lie on the back, and the covering should be light and the bed hard. When patients

awake in the morning they should at once empty the bladder.

The treatment of sexual neurasthenia in general, means the correction of general nerve depression. Aside from local treatment, which may be necessary when strictures or old discharges complicate the trouble, or when a tight prepuce exists or rectal irritation from piles or retained fecal matter, the essential object always, is the relief of nerve-depression on which the sexual disorders are dependent. Charlatans often aggravate the sexual weakness and irritability by employing drugs and different kinds of apparatus, which temporarily stimulate the debilitated organs, leaving them in a worse condition than ever before. In no other disease is meddlesome treatment so disastrous as in sexual debility, and many individuals have been permanently injured by such measures. There are no specific drugs in the treatment of sexual neurasthenia. Even moral treatment, so often vaunted by medical writers, is of little avail, and while the mind frequently operates to the disadvantage of the sexual apparatus, there is no affection which is less amenable to moral treatment than sexual neurasthenia. Patients see no results in expectancy. They want results, and the results which they are so eager to obtain can only be achieved by a correct toning of the nervous system.

HYPNOTISM.

Treatment by suggestion, when intelligently employed in neurasthenia, is capable of marvelous effects in ridding the patient of morbid ideas and in inducing sleep, which, even with drugs, is often impossible.

Healthy suggestions made by the physician, I regard

as indispensable in the treatment of many cases. The dangers of hypnotism are exaggerated, for no one can be hypnotized against his wish. Prof. Bernheim, the apostle of hypnotism, has this to say: " It is the duty of the physician to select what is useful in suggestion, and to apply it for the benefit of his patients. When, in the presence of sickness, I think that therapeutic suggestion has a chance of success, I should consider myself to blame, as a physician, if I did not propose it to my patient, and if I did not even make a point of getting his consent to its employment." The influence of the mind on the body is every day illustrated by the introduction of some new fad or delusion in the treatment of disease. It is difficult to conceive that such results are effected by the mind as a simple thinking organ; on the contrary, the mind is psychodynamic, and must be regarded as a force like light, heat and electricity which operates for good or evil on the bodily functions. Strong mental impressions may actuate disease, and even death, or they may act by curing disease. Joy and hope stimulate, whereas grief and despair depress the bodily functions. Sutton presents the following facts, which are apposite in this connection:

FIRST. That mental emotion may induce sickness or death within a brief space of time, or even immediately, and in persons of robust health.

SECOND. The physical phenomena induced by such cause indicate a deep perturbation—vibration—of the nervous system, and are generally of a dynamic character.

THIRD. Thought strongly directed to any part tends to increase its vascularity and consequently its sensibility.

FOURTH. Thought strongly directed away from any part diminishes vascularity and lessens sensibility. The more so when associated with powerful emotions. (A key which unlocks Christian science and other " fads.")

FIFTH. The emotions may cause sensations, either by directly exciting the sensory ganglia and the central extremities of the nerves of sensation, or by inducing vascular changes in a certain part of the body, which excite the sensitive nerves at their peripheral termination.

SIXTH. There is no sensation, whether general or special, excited by agents acting on the body from without, which cannot be excited also from within by emotional states affecting the sensory ganglia, such sensation being referred by the mind to the point at which the nerve terminates in the body. (Tuke.)

Christian Science is suggestion plus absurdity; divine healing, suggestion plus faith in God; Dowieism, suggestion plus prayer and holy terror; Weltmerism, suggestion plus imagination, pure; magnetic healing, suggestion plus imagination, also; osteopathy, suggestion plus massage; homeopathy, suggestion plus nothing; allopathy, suggestion plus tubfuls of drugs that either kill or cure; regular or rational medicine, suggestion plus the best common horse sense available, or suggestion and medicine mixed with the best quality of brains obtainable. No suggestion in this that the quality of brains is indisputably good in all cases—or perhaps in any. Yet that is the scientific principle at the base, and it may be used with telling effect in all cases of sickness, and is infinitely better than the delusions of the day by so much as it substitutes intelligence for ignorance and does not produce that disaggregation of personal consciousness and temporary insanity that is the *sine qua non* in Christian Science, etc.

There are many competent writers who doubt the utility of hypnotism in therapeutics and aver that its results are achieved at the expense of demoralization. My own observations with hypnotism as a therapeutic agent extending over a period of fifteen years justify me in the conclusion, that when judiciously employed in carefully selected cases, it is a most effective agent, and results may be attained which are incapable of achievement by any other known means. The latter statement refers not only to disease, but also of education for the improvement of character and morals. It was supposed at one time that only weak, sick, nervous and hysterical women were susceptible to hypnotism, but the extensive statistics of Liébault have shown that almost anybody can be hypnotized, the susceptibility to suggestion being influenced by willingness of the subject, his passivity and the power to concentrate the thought or attention on the intended sleep. Intelligent persons are more difficult subjects than mechanics or laborers, because they permit their thoughts, whether voluntary or involuntary, to wander to various objects which distract the attention. Patience and renewed seances are often rewarded by success in those who are not susceptible to the influence. Young are more susceptible than old persons, and women more easily influenced than men.

SUMMARY.

1. Reliance on the healing power of Nature is an evidence of erudition. It affords the discerning physician an opportunity of knowing what not to do, a feat often more difficult than doing, and enables him to apply the highest principles of the therapeutic art.

2. "The confession and absolution of sanitary sins is a constant physical force in medical practice. The physician is the priest of health; his gospel is the one of right living." (Dr. H. C. Sawyer.)

3. "The attitude of a patient should be that of a voyager who resigns himself to the captain, and does not look for the further shore until the time comes." (Beard.)

4. "There is wisdom in this beyond the rules of physic. A man's own observation, what he finds good and of what he finds hurt of, is the best physic to preserve health." (Bacon.)

5. "We are all prone to forget—that we are dealing with human beings whose hopes and fears are played upon by our every word and act as subtly as the most wonderful musical instrument is touched by the fingers of the master performer. We may thus be the creators of the sweetest strains of human feeling, or the insensible performers upon sweet bells jangled out of tune." (Dr. Geo. M. Gould.)

6. "A physician whose horizon is bounded by an historical knowledge of the human machine, and who can only distinguish terminologically and locally, the coarser wheels of this piece of intellectual clock-work, may perhaps be idolized by the mob, but he will never

raise the Hippocratic art above the narrow sphere of a mere bread-earning craft." (Schiller.)

7. " Any physician who neglects to approach physical symptoms through the mind will find the practice of medicine a sorry task. The physician is often compelled to conciliate the mind of the patient while Nature is effecting the cure.

8. " To eat little, and that little of simple food, is to prolong life." (Cornaro.)

9. " For my part, when I see a fashionable table set out in all its magnificence, I fancy I see gouts and dropsies, fears and innumerable distempers lying in ambuscade among the dishes." (Addison.)

10. " Good ventilation and a certain amount of out-of-door bodily exercise are of the greatest importance and greatest necessity in insuring good, refreshing sleep, as well as a good old age." (Hufeland.)

11. " Those are greatly mistaken who believe that a modern physician is he who examines a patient most carefully, auscultates and percusses, and is satisfied when the autopsy corresponds with his diagnosis. Such a medical man does not comprehend that the aim of all medical service is the healing of the sick." (Oppolzer.)

12. " Pathology is the physiology of the sick." (Wunderlich.)

13. " Let me diet a person and I can give him almost any kind of disease known,—long life or short life." (Dr. T. R. Allison.)

14. " Medicine has taken possession of hypnotism, and it is only through her that such an agent can be made of use to mankind and prevented from working injury to the human race." (Charcot.)

15. Decalogue of Health (Dr. Frank H. Hamilton):

" 1. The best thing for the inside of a man is the outside of a horse."

"2. Blessed is he who invented sleep—but thrice blessed the man who will invent a cure for thinking.

" 3. Light gives a bronzed or tan color to the skin; but where it uproots the lily it plants the rose.

" 4. The lives of most men are in their own hands, and, as a rule, the just verdict after death would be—*felo de se*.

" 5. Health must be earned—it can seldom be bought.

" 6. A change of air is less valuable than a change of scene. The air is changed every time the wind is changed.

" 7. Mold and decaying vegetables in a cellar weave shrouds for the upper chambers.

" 8. Dirt, debauchery, disease, and death are successive links in the same chain.

" 9. Calisthenics may be very genteel, and romping very ungenteel, but one is the shadow, the other the substance, of healthful exercise.

" 10. Girls need health as much—nay, more than boys. They can only obtain it as boys do, by running, tumbling—by all sorts of innocent vagrancy. At least once a day girls should have their halters taken off, the bars let down, and be turned loose like young colts.

" 11. The alimentary regimen in neurasthenia is important, for neurasthenics eat too much. The amount of food consumed should be reduced to what is absolutely necessary and this is gauged by weight and strength. If the latter, grow less, the amount of food taken must be increased. Neurasthenics eat too much, but do not drink enough. At least 3 pints of water should be advised for daily consumption. Digestion always means an expenditure of nerve force, therefore it is wise to remember that a minimum of food means a minimum of digestive work. The foregoing facts are specially applicable in splanchnic neurasthenia.

"12. I believe it was Carlyle, who said 'that the average American meal was an unpunished crime.' Nervous dyspeptics should not indulge in regulation meals, but should eat often. This rule, if followed, will reduce the task of a stomach suddenly overburdened with food and will diminish the tendency to overeat.

"13. The recent experiments of Prof. Anderson, of Yale University, prove that the most important thing in all exercises is the mental effort put forth. Exercises if conducted automatically, will not divert the blood as they should from the brain to the muscles. Prof. Gates, was able, by thinking intently of one of his hands, when it was immersed in a basin full of water, and willing that the blood should flow there, to make the water overflow. The foregoing facts are sold by teachers of physical culture for good prices and they emphasize that very little exercise, with the mind directing it, will effectually rebuild the body."

CHAPTER VI.

SPLANCHNIC NEURASTHENIA.

THE BLUES.

WHY THE TERM, " THE BLUES," HAS BEEN EMPLOYED TO SPECIFY THIS PARTICULAR FORM OF NEURASTHENIA. —DATA BEARING ON SPLANCHNIC NEURASTHENIA.— INTRA-ABDOMINAL PRESSURE, PULMONARY SUCTION, VASOMOTOR FACTOR.—THE ABDOMINAL SYMPATHETIC. —FACTORS CONTRIBUTING TO SPLANCHNIC NEURAS-THENIA.

SPLANCHNIC NEURASTHENIA is, above all things, characterized by attacks of *depression*, which come on spontaneously without apparent cause and depart as mysteriously as they came. The subjects of such attacks specify their condition at the time as " *a fit of the blues.*" " The blues," occur usually in neurasthenic individuals, and, being of short duration, in most instances, may be spoken of technically as attacks of acute neurasthenia. Not infrequently, they may be of prolonged duration, in which instances, they may be referred to as exacerbations of chronic neurasthenia. To clearly comprehend splanchnic neurasthenia, it will be necessary to direct our attention to the abdomen and restrict consideration to *intra-abdominal tension* and the effects of such tension on the blood circulation in the abdomen.

INTRA-ABDOMINAL TENSION. This refers to the pressure in the abdominal cavity. In the normal subject, the pressure is positive, that is, it is greater than the atmospheric pressure, hence the abdominal walls are pressed outward. Tension within the abdomen is chiefly dependent on the contraction of the abdominal walls, and this in turn is dependent on the strength of the muscles which make up the abdominal walls. In other words, when the abdominal muscles are strong, all other things being equal, intra-abdominal tension is increased, and when they are feeble, the same tension is decreased.

FACTORS WHICH INCREASE AND DECREASE INTRA-ABDOMINAL PRESSURE.

The tone of the anterior abdominal muscles is *increased* in certain occupations which tend to develop them. Thus, the strong, hard, flat abdomens of fishermen who fish with nets and spend many hours dragging at the ropes may be contrasted with the protruding bellies of shoemakers and tailors, in whom an insufficient development of the muscles occurs, owing to their relaxation, the result of posture in their special occupations. Tension is *diminished,* when fat accumulates in the walls of the abdomen, in corset-wearing women and chiefly as a result of pregnancy. Schwerdt,[22] refers to reduced intra-abdominal pressure as a result of relaxation of the whole nervous system, which reacts on the muscular system. Other factors concerned in the reduction of tension are: 1. Hereditary factors; 2. Mental overwork; 3. Insufficient nourishment; 4. Chronic diseases. According to Glenard,[23] diminution of the intra-abdominal tension is due more to the lessening of the volume of gas in the intestines than to any other cause. That this latter cause is important, I will endeavor to show later, but I do not accept the view of Glenard, viz.: that intra-abdominal tension is the expression of the forces which regulate the relationship between the capacity of the abdominal cavity and the volume of its contents. When the abdominal walls atrophy, the intestines fill with gas.

EFFECTS OF DIMINISHED INTRA-ABDOMINAL TENSION. The positive pressure exerted by the tonic contraction of the anterior abdominal muscles is probably the most important factor in keeping the abdominal organs in place, for when they are relaxed as a permanent condition, their pressure on the underlying structures is insufficient and the result is, a dislocation of. the organs. This particular function of abdominal tension, while an important one, merits little consideration in developing our particular subject, viz.: splanchnic neurasthenia. While it is true, that dislocation of the abdominal organs is associated with a very intractable form of neurasthenia, with preponderance of abdominal symptoms; in splanchnic neurasthenia, dislocation of the abdominal organs has been an infrequent phenomenon in my experience, and when present, was only indirectly concerned in the nervous symptoms. In fact, in dislocation of the abdominal organs, the development of subsequent nervous symptoms is due largely to the effects on the *abdominal circulation,* and this, together with ptosis of the viscera, is only an effect of diminished intra-abdominal tension.

EFFECTS OF REDUCED INTRA-ABDOMINAL TENSION ON THE CIRCULATION. This is the most important factor concerned in splanchnic neurasthenia, and has received scant consideration from physicians, a most la-

8

mentable fact, considering the gravity of the issues involved. Tension within the abdominal cavity directly influences the blood circulation in the abdominal organs, digestive functions and indirectly almost every organ of the body. The abdominal veins are very capacious, and experiments have taught, that they are capable of holding all the blood in the body. The amount of blood in the abdominal or splanchnic veins is merely a question of abdominal tension. When the latter is diminished, the veins contain more blood than when the tension is increased. Hill and Barnard,[24] have contributed largely to this important subject in a physiologic direction, and Campbell,[25] has sought to elaborate it practically. They have demonstrated that there is a tendency of the blood to accumulate in the splanchnic area, with consequent syncope. Like the generality of veins, the great splanchnic veins are very susceptible to pressure, and the amount of blood within them is greatly influenced by pressure of the abdominal walls. Mere pressure of the abdomen suffices to squeeze out of the veins a large quantity of blood. Thus gravity, posture, the accoutrements of dress and other factors greatly influence the amount of blood contained in the abdominal veins. More blood accumulates in the veins in the erect than in the recumbent posture, and it is not an uncommon observation for syncope to occur in bedridden patients, who are suddenly constrained to get out of bed. The removal of stays in women often induces a feeling of faintness, and the same symptom may occur in susceptible persons when the bladder is voided or the feces discharged. Three factors enter into consideration in the mechanism of blood supply to the splanchnic vessels, viz.: 1. The contraction of the abdominal muscles; 2. The act of respiration; 3. The regulating vasomotor action of the splanchnic vessels.

THE ABDOMINAL FACTOR. The transversales muscles maintain the anterior posterior abdominal walls in fairly close contact, and prevent, in the erect posture, gravitation of the blood into the splanchnic veins.

THE RESPIRATORY FACTOR. That important muscle of respiration, the diaphragm, acts in opposition to the abdominal muscles. Weakness of the abdominal muscles signifies a weak diaphragm. When the latter contracts, it has to work against the intra-abdominal pressure, which it increases, hence, if abdominal pressure is reduced by weakened abdominal muscles, the diaphragm has little work to perform and consequently its strength diminishes. Every time the diaphragm descends, the intra-abdominal vessels are compressed, and the action thus exerted is less evident in the tense arteries than in the flaccid veins; the blood being squeezed out of the latter into the right chambers of the heart. De Jager [26] has shown, that even strong pressure upon the abdomen has little or no effect on the arteries, but serves to squeeze a large quantity of blood from the splanchnic veins. Hill has also shown that, in consequence of some failure, in certain compensatory mechanisms, the blood gravitates into the splanchnic veins from the right heart and that pressure upon the abdomen will send back the blood from these veins to the right heart, and thus re-establish the circulation.

PULMONARY SUCTION refers to the large quantity of blood drawn into the lungs with each inspiration, and this physiologic process has not been inaptly compared to a species of dry cupping. Chapman [27] avers, " That if at the termination of expiration the quantity of blood in the lungs is from 1-15 to 1-18 of the total quantity of blood in the body, at the termination of inspiration, it will be from 1-12 to 1-13." The pulmonary vessels expand with each inspiration and contract during expiration, the result being an increased flow of blood from the right heart and the lungs; the dilated vessels, as Campbell[28] puts it, " actually suck the blood out of the right heart."

VASOMOTOR FACTOR. The splanchnic nerves possess the power of regulating the amount of blood in the splanchnic veins, and prevent the gravitation of blood into them.

The quantity of blood, which may be forced by abdominal pressure into the heart, and from thence into the general circulation, has never been determined objectively until I directed attention to what I have called the " Cardio-Splanchnic Phenomenon." * It was this phenomenon which enabled me to appreciate the tendency of blood to gravitate into the abdominal veins in many neurasthenics, and to inhibit the symptoms of the latter by treatment directed against this tendency. Before elaborating the phenomena which contribute to this special form of neurasthenia, I wish briefly to direct attention to the nerve apparatus, which presides over the function of innervation of the organs contained in the abdominal cavity, viz.: the abdominal sympathetic.

THE ABDOMINAL SYMPATHETIC. The relations of the great sympathetic with the cerebro-spinal axis, and the nature of its functions is a matter involved in much obscurity. This much we do know, however, that it exerts an important influence over the circulation, secretions and nutrition of the organs innervated by it. In

* See Appendix, Note 2.

health, the abdominal sympathetic confers an uncon-
scious sensibility to the abdominal organs, but when irritated from any cause, violent pains and abnormal sensations are experienced, not only at the point of irritation, but reflexly, owing to its communication with
branches of the cerebro-spinal system of nerves, at remote situations. Irritation of the splanchnic nerves is
attended primarily by contraction of the abdominal
vessels, but the latter soon dilate, leading to a stagnation of blood. Byron Robinson [29] refers to the celiac
ganglia, the largest in the body, as the ABDOMINAL
BRAIN, which acts as a reflex center outside of the
spinal cord.

Meinert [30] claims that the celiac plexus controls the
formation of hemoglobin in the spleen. The coats of all
the principal blood-vessels in the abdomen are supplied
by the sympathetic nerve, which regulates the vascular
supply to the organs.

FACTORS WHICH CONTRIBUTE TO THE DEVELOP-
MENT OF SPLANCHNIC NEURASTHENIA.

This form of neurasthenia is dependent essentially on
a stagnation of the blood in the splanchnic or abdominal
veins. This is the primary and fundamental condition
prevailing in splanchnic neurasthenia. The factors
which conduce to this condition are many, but in most
instances, it is lack of nerve force exerted through the
muscles of the abdomen and respiration and the nervous
mechanism which regulates the supply of blood in the
veins. From this, one would be constrained to conclude,
that the phenomenon of blood stagnation in the abdominal veins is not a primary but a condition secondary
to nervous exhaustion. In this contention, one would be

partially correct, for, while it is usually a secondary condition, it is not infrequently a primary one. It is capable of aggravating a neurasthenic disposition, and induces it when absent. By treatment directed toward the stagnation of blood in the abdominal veins, I have succeeded in curing many neurasthenics of their vicious symptoms, notably, mental depression and of limiting their fatigue signs to the sphere to which they properly belong, the brain and spinal cord. This is practically all that can be accomplished for the neurasthenic by the physician. The fatigue symptoms of the former are the result of his own indiscretion, and his mastery of them presumes sufficient intelligence, which enables him to recognize his own power of endurance.

NERVE FORCE LACKING IN THE MUSCLES OF THE ABDOMEN. I have already shown that the greater intra-abdominal tension, the less blood will be contained in the abdominal veins. Furthermore, that this tension is largely dependent on the tone or tension of the abdominal muscles. Now, tone in any muscle or group of muscles is the product of a storm of nervous impulses pouring into them from a nerve center, and when the latter is fatigued, the tone of the muscle diminishes, which is expressed by relaxation of the muscular fibers. Therefore, nervous exhaustion is a frequent cause of diminished tone of the abdominal muscles, which in turn diminishes intra-abdominal tension, and conduces to blood stagnation in the veins of the abdomen.

NERVE FORCE LACKING IN THE FUNCTION OF RESPIRATION. Here, as in the preceding condition, the same cause prevails. Not only in neurasthenia, but in other functional nervous diseases, respiratory exercises have been shown to be of great value. This effect, to my

THE CAUSE AND CURE.

mind, has been achieved through their influence on the
abdominal circulation. The lungs are important avenues for the elimination of poisonous substances, many
of which are scarcely known. By healthy lung action,
we may regulate the local and general blood and lymph
circulations. Such effects are not only local, but general, for every protoplasmic unit of the body to live
must have its essential quantity of oxygen, and receiving
this, yields in return its products of activity. We have
already referred to " pulmonary suction," showing how,
with each inspiration, the blood is sucked, as it were,
from the veins throughout the body, and this, in reference to the abdominal veins constitutes an important
factor in diminishing venous turgescence in the abdominal cavity. The flow of blood is urged primarily into
the cavæ and right heart, from the latter into the lungs,
and from the latter into the left heart. In other words,
depletion of the veins is accomplished by forcible respiration, so that the supply to the arteries is thereby
increased, and nutrition of the tissues and organs facili-
tated. The question of *blood pressure,* as a result of
compression of the abdomen, is referred to in the appendix.* There is another factor concerned in respiration, which bears on the venous circulation in the abdominal cavity, and that is, the descent of the diaphragm. Every time the latter muscle descends in inspiration, it increases intra-abdominal tension, and ex-
presses a considerable amount of blood out of the intra-
abdominal veins into the right heart. The action of
the diaphragm in effecting this object is dependent on
the condition of the abdominal walls: if they are vigorous, intra-abdominal tension is increased, and the

* See Appendix, Note 8.

quantity of blood squeezed out of the veins is correspondingly augmented; if the abdominal walls are relaxed, there is little or no effect on the intra-abdominal tension, nor on the intra-abdominal veins.

NERVE FORCE LACKING IN THE NERVOUS MECHANISM WHICH REGULATES THE SUPPLY OF BLOOD IN THE ABDOMINAL VEINS. The *vasomotor nervous system* supplies the muscular tissue in the walls of the blood-vessels and regulates their caliber. Ordinarily, the small arteries are maintained in a state of moderate or tonic contraction, which is necessary to force the blood in a continuous stream through the capillaries and veins back to the heart. Another function exercised by this system is to regulate the amount of blood which flows through the capillaries of any organ in proportion to its needs. Thus, during digestion, it is imperative that there should be a large quantity of blood supplied to the digestive organs, hence at this time, the small arteries of the splanchnic area are relaxed, and there is a large amount of blood in this area, and a corresponding small amount in other areas, such as the skin, and it is for this reason that sensations of chilliness are experienced after a capacious meal. Splanchnic neurasthenics for a similar reason experience an intensification of their symptoms after a full meal, for it is at this time that the abdominal organs are surcharged with blood. The most important vasomotor nerves of the body are the splanchnics, with their cell stations situated in the various ganglia of the abdominal plexuses. Now, in many cases of neurasthenia (*Angiopathic neurasthenia*) the vasomotor symptoms are extremely prominent, and it would seem as if the nerve exhaustion in such cases were mainly resident in the vasomotor system.

RECAPITULATION. Reviewing the factors concerned in splanchnic neurasthenia, we may deduce the following: Defective innervation from any cause leads to congestion of the abdominal veins; Venous congestion interferes with a proper supply of arterial blood; The tissues and organs bathed in pools of stagnant blood are practically in a state of asphyxia; The toxic products of digestion, which are normally removed by an unimpeded circulation, have a specifically poisonous effect on the sympathetic system, a fact which is evident, owing to the frequent occurrence of depression, prostration and nervous symptoms in nearly all disorders of the alimentary canal. Venous congestion diminishes the vital tone of the organs and lessens their vital resistance. This subject will be further elaborated in the next chapter on the symptoms of splanchnic neurasthenia.

SUMMARY.

1.   Depression is one of the most important symptoms of splanchnic neurasthenia, hence the layman is prone to specify his sensations as a " fit of the blues."

2.   " A fit of the blues " is, technically speaking, acute neurasthenia, but it may also be an aggravated paroxysm of chronic neurasthenia.

3.   The entire question of splanchnic neurasthenia is one of abdominal plethora, dependent on a variety of causes, notably, diminished intra-abdominal tension, insufficient lung development, and a defective vasomotor apparatus.

4.   The foregoing causes are dependent in a great measure on diminished nerve tone, which seeks the foregoing avenues for expression.

5.   Splanchnic neurasthenia is one of the few forms of neurasthenia amenable to permanent cure by measures having for their object the relief of abdominal venous congestion.

6.   Intra-abdominal venous congestion is tantamount to asphyxiation of the abdominal viscera with all its evil consequences.

CHAPTER VII.

THE SYMPTOMS OF SPLANCHNIC NEURASTHENIA.

HISTORY OF A SPLANCHNIC NEURASTHENIC.—ANALYSIS
OF THE MOST PROMINENT SYMPTOMS.—RELAXED AB-
DOMINAL WALLS, PROTRUSION OF THE ABDOMEN.—
GAS ACCUMULATION IN THE BOWELS, INCREASED AB-
DOMINAL TENDERNESS, ENLARGEMENT OF THE LIVER,
AND INSUFFICIENT LUNG DEVELOPMENT.

I WILL introduce this subject by presenting, in detail,
the history of a patient, the subject of *splanchnic neurasthenia,* after which, I will submit to analysis the
most prominent symptoms.

HISTORY OF A CASE OF SPLANCHNIC NEURASTHENIA.
The patient is an attorney, age 35. He presents no definite history of excesses of any kind. For the past three
years he has become exceedingly irritable, and has what
he calls *" blue streaks,"* which come on at irregular intervals without any apparent cause, although he is inclined to the belief that he can nearly always trace their
origin to some error in diet. What this error is, he does
not know; it is not any particular kind of food, but it
may be a late supper or a meal eaten hastily. At any
rate, during his " blue streaks," he has *uncomfortable
abdominal sensations,* which he is unable to describe
fully. Although his bowels move regularly during his
" blue periods," they are inclined to looseness. His

" blue streaks " have become more frequent of late, and last longer. Intense mental *depression* and *prostration* attend the attacks. At such times he is incapable of doing work. He wants to be left severely alone during . the attacks. Of late, his *memory* has become affected, and he is unable to concentrate his attention. He lacks decision in his mental operations and control. He has *morbid fancies.* He thinks that death would be a happy release from his suffering, and constantly dwells on the subject of self-destruction. In the intervals of his attacks, which have become less and less frequent, he never has the sensation of well-being. He can no longer pursue his vocation with the same buoyancy as before, in fact, he works automatically. His symptoms are *intensified after eating,* and for an hour or so, after a meal, he becomes horribly depressed and irritable. He has no symptoms of indigestion in the ordinary sense, but large quantities of *gas accumulate in the bowels.* For a time, he practically starved himself, so that he could be released from the depression and irritability following meals. He has submitted himself to all kinds of treatment without relief. One physician had treated him for *uric acid neurasthenia,* and at that time he experienced temporary relief. My examination revealed in brief the following: *Imperfect lung development, feeble heart action, protrusion of the abdomen with gas accumulation in the bowels, exquisite sensitiveness of the abdomen, enlargement of the liver,* which was extremely painful on pressure, and the *abdominal walls* were relaxed and showed no tone. Removal of the stomach contents after a test meal demonstrated no anomaly.

This is in brief, the typical history of a case of *splanchnic neurasthenia.*

The objective signs will primarily merit our consideration.

THE ABDOMINAL WALLS. Relaxation of the abdominal walls is a common objective sign in this form of neurasthenia. The abdomen is normally flat, and remains so in health until the end of life. In some, especially women, a hanging belly is best observed when the patient assumes the erect posture. In the horizontal position, the abdomen flattens and bulges at the sides. The skin of the abdomen is loose, and this, together with the flaccid walls, allows not only easy palpitation of the underlying organs, but they may sometimes be seen. Feeble abdominal muscles may be concealed by a large deposit of fat, but the condition of the muscles may be fairly gauged by directing the patient to raise the body while lying supine or to bear down forcibly, when the vigor of muscular contraction can be estimated by the fingers. In pronounced cases, there is a wide space between the abdominal recti. Another method of testing relaxed abdominal walls is to stand behind the patient, place the hands at each side of the abdomen and then, drawing the abdomen wall toward you, suddenly release it; the degree of relaxation is determined by the distance which the abdominal wall falls after its release. Stiller [31] referred to a sign which was present in a large number of neurasthenics, specially those who were lean and dyspeptic, and that was, a *mobile tenth rib,* which was not fixed with the cartilage to the other ribs, but was either wholly free (or floating) or attached only with ligament. This " Costa fluctuans decima " is, according to him, very common in delicate children and that they are apt to become neurasthenics or enteroptotics later in life, according as nervous or dyspeptic symptoms predominate.

Our main object in testing relaxation of the abdominal wall in splanchnic neurasthenia is really to determine how far such relaxation comprises the intra-abdominal venous circulation, and for this purpose reference is made to the *cardio-splanchnic phenomenon*.* The more the latter is in evidence, as determined by the degree of dulness and the extent of its area, the more pronounced will be the circulatory embarrassment.

PROTRUSION OF THE ABDOMEN. This occurs, as a rule, owing to diminished intra-abdominal pressure on the intestines, which allows their readier distension with gas with consequent pressure effects on the abdominal wall.

GAS ACCUMULATION IN THE BOWELS. This is a frequent symptom, and, which I hope to show, is one of compensation. The accumulation of gas in the intestines increases intra-abdominal tension, and any increase in the latter means diminished intra-abdominal venous congestion. The gases of the intestinal canal are derived in part from the air (oxygen and nitrogen), in part from the ingesta (carbonic acid) and in part from intestinal fermentation (ammonia, carbonic acid, hydrogen, hydrogen sulphide, etc.). Some of the gas is removed by eructations and by flatus, as well as through resorption by the blood-vessels, as is evidenced by the increased excretion of carbonic acid through the lungs, occurring usually about an hour after a meal. In the chemistry of respiration, the air in the lungs and the blood in the capillaries are separated only by the thin capillaries and alveolar walls. The blood parts with its excess of

* Appendix, Note 2.

carbonic acid to the air in the lungs, and the blood simultaneously engages the oxygen from the air in the lungs. This intake of oxygen and output of carbonic acid takes place all over the body, and constitutes what is called *tissue-respiration*. If we apply this theory to the congested abdominal veins, we have the following: The intestines and abdominal veins represent two chambers containing a mixture of gases in unequal amount; diffusion takes place until the percentage amount of each gas in each chamber is the same. Owing to the stagnation of blood in the abdominal veins, the latter contain a large quantity of carbonic acid, hence carbonic acid diffuses from the veins to the intestines. The intestines now being inflated, increase intra-abdominal tension, which in turn squeezes the blood out of the abdominal veins to the right heart. After this manner, gas accumulation in the intestines, is, as I view it, distinctly a compensatory process, and the results attained by treatment justify this conclusion. Gas accumulation in the intestines in splanchnic neurasthenia gives rise to many symptoms, especially referable to the heart.*

INCREASED SENSITIVENESS OF THE ABDOMEN.*

Splanchnic neurasthenics, as a rule, are very susceptible to pressure made on the anterior abdominal wall. The abdomen may be diffusely sensitive on deep pressure or the sensitive points may be localized, and remind one of the hysterogenic zones. The site of predilection of the sensitive points is the lower abdomen. Not infrequently pains radiate to the back, to the neck and to the legs, and may be of the most agonizing character. The

* Appendix, Note 4.
* Appendix, Note 11.

pains in question do not admit of localization with reference to any nerve trunk, or its terminal distribution, and they are not modified by pressure, rest nor movement.   These facts suggest the abdominal origin of the pains which are probably caused by congestion of the intra-abdominal veins irritating *the terminal ramifications* of the *splanchnic nerves.*   There is one fact worthy of mention in diagnosis with reference to abdominal sensitiveness and liver tenderness, and that is, if firm compression of the abdomen is made with the hands and the process repeated for several minutes, abdominal sensitiveness, liver tenderness and the radiating pains become markedly abated and even disappear after several minutes.   The phenomenon in question is clearly the result of the maneuver, and receives the following explanation: Abdominal compression will squeeze the blood out of the intra-abdominal veins, and will thus remove the source of irritation acting on the splanchnic nerves.

ENLARGEMENT OF THE LIVER.*   This is an almost invariable accompaniment of splanchnic neurasthenia. Aside from enlargement, the liver is always palpable, and found to be exquisitely painful.   It is more painful after eating, and the sensation of fullness experienced after a meal by splanchnic neurasthenics is frequently caused by hepatic *engorgement.*   This hepatic tenderness is always associated with neurasthenic symptoms, and is always more pronounced when the latter are intensified.   After a night's rest, the hepatic tenderness is no longer evident in the morning, but soon after breakfast it reappears and becomes more marked as the day proceeds, increasing in severity after each meal.   Hepatic enlargement and tenderness may be made to dis-

* Appendix ; Note 5.

appear in most instances by vigorous massage of the abdomen and the application of the sinusoidal current, facts which will be elaborated in the chapter on the special treatment of splanchnic neurasthenia. The sinusoidal current induces what I have called the *liver reflex.** The liver has from time immemorial been surreptitiously accused of participation in an attack of " the blues," and, for want of a better term, " biliousness " has heretofore been employed to designate the condition. I have frequently examined individuals during an attack of " the blues," and have established the fact to my own satisfaction that hepatic enlargement and tenderness accompany the paroxysm. Furthermore, that treatment having for its object the depletion of the intra-abdominal veins will abort an attack or diminish its severity. In what way does the liver participate in the attacks in question ? The amount of blood which the liver contains has been estimated by Foster [32] to be equivalent to one-fourth the amount of blood contained in the body. The blood is chiefly derived from the portal vein, which collects blood from the stomach, intestine, spleen and pancreas. Digestion increases the amount of blood contained in the intra-abdominal veins (*physiologic congestion*), a fact which accounts for the drowsiness felt by some dyspeptics soon after eating, the result of brain anemia from portal congestion. The cold extremities of some dyspeptics during the digestive stage admit of the same explanation.

My investigations show that coincident with this congestion of the intra-abdominal veins after meals there is a corresponding rise in the blood pressure which is most pronounced one hour after meals, then it gradually falls

* Appendix: Note 6.

9

until the next meal time. It is this increased blood
pressure after meals which aggravates the condition of
the splanchnic neurasthenic at such particular periods,
the augmented blood pressure injuring the delicate tissues of the brain by a series of powerful uniform blows,
and one is justified in referring to such action as, *the
traumatism of high blood pressure.*

Now, the secretion of the bile is effected by stimulation of the liver cell by digestive products carried to the
liver. Aside from the many established functions of the
liver, experiment and pathology demonstrate that the
liver is endowed with the function of not only arresting
but of destroying toxic substances which are developed
in the ordinary process of digestion and from intestinal
putrefaction. It is not difficult to understand, then, why
it is, that in splanchnic neurasthenia, hepatic tenderness
and enlargement are worse after eating, and why it is,
that in this affection, mental depression and prostration
are such prominent symptoms: They are clearly the
result of *auto-intoxication;* the functions of the liver
being inhibited by congestion and the toxic products
from the intestinal canal being no longer arrested nor
destroyed pass into the circulation inducing pronounced
nervous symptoms, of which mental depression and prostration are the most prominent. If there are periods
during the day in which nervous symptoms remit in
splanchnic neurasthenia, such periods occur several
hours after eating. Thus, in splanchnic neurasthenia,
the " fatigue curve " is not always identical with that
which occurs in neurasthenia, the result of overwork.
In the latter form of the affection, the ebb of nerve force
begins with the early morning hours, attains its maximum discharge in the middle of the afternoon, when the

nervously exhausted are most weak. Many splanchnic
neurasthenics have and are being treated for a supposi-
titious *uric acid intoxication.* Whatever organ may be
accredited with the manufacture of uric acid or the nature of the symptoms produced by the latter, this much
is evident, that uric acid does no more in explaining
gout than it does the nervous symptoms supposed to be
attributed to it, but it hints at defective hepatic meta-
bolism, or as Yeo [38] would call it, " *hepatic inadequacy.*"
In other words, there is some disturbance in function
antecedent to the accumulation of uric acid in the blood
which is responsible for gout, rheumatism, neurasthenia
and a multitude of allied affections. Experiments suggest the theory that urea and uric acid are formed in
the liver,[84] and admitting, for the sake of argument,
that uric acid is responsible for the preceding affections,
and that the source of its production is in the liver, reasoning by analogy, this conclusion is warranted: that
an organ in a healthy state which produces any substance can also repress that substance when its over-
production is inimical to the integrity of the economy.
Approaching the final signs, which I have frequently
encountered in splanchnic neurasthenia, we have insufficient lung development and heart weakness.

INSUFFICIENT LUNG DEVELOPMENT. Diminished
intra-abdominal tension implies reduced strength of the
diaphragm, and the elimination of this powerful muscle
in respiration seriously compromises lung development,
hence, in splanchnic neurasthenia, the lungs fail to perform the work required of them, and another factor is
added to further embarrass the already imperfect abdominal circulation.

HEART WEAKNESS. Here many factors conspire to

bring about heart weakness. First, stagnation of blood
in the abdomen means an insufficient blood supply to the
heart; second, there is a deficient supply of oxygen in
the blood (Anoxemia), and the heart, like every tissue,
suffers; third, the toxic substances present in the blood
reduce the vital tone of the heart, and the resistance of
the latter, like every other organ in the body, is necessarily reduced. In concluding this chapter, I wish to
emphasize the very important fact, that splanchnic neurasthenia may exist without the appreciation of any
abdominal symptoms by the patient; and on the other
hand, while the local abdominal symptoms may be slight,
the reflex symptoms may be so pronounced that they
compromise the integrity of all the organs including the
nervous system, the heart, the alimentary canal and the
sexual organs.

SUMMARY.

1.   The dominant symptoms of splanchnic neurasthenia are resident in the nervous system.

2.   Many splanchnic neurasthenics are never cognizant of abdominal symptoms; the latter being usually elicited by the physician in the course of his examination.

3.   The chief abdominal symptoms are: Abdominal sensitiveness, tenderness of the liver and enlargement of that organ and gaseous accumulation in the bowels.

4.   It is often difficult to say how much of the nervousness in the average neurasthenic is due to intra-abdominal venous congestion, for the latter condition may aggravate the symptoms of neurasthenia. The only test is the therapeutic one: by eliminating the venous element, which is certainly possible of achievement, we may observe the effect on the nervous symptoms.

5.   In splanchnic neurasthenia existing as an independent affection, the relief of symptoms almost positively follows relief of the venous abdominal congestion.

6.   The Cardio-splanchnic phenomenon is a trustworthy index of the severity of the affection, and in gauging the results of treatment.

7.   Splanchnic neurasthenia is specially encountered in individuals with vigorous constitutions, in whom the question of an unhygienic life does not enter into consideration. Nor can the conventional factors always be elicited in the history which conduce to neurasthenia.

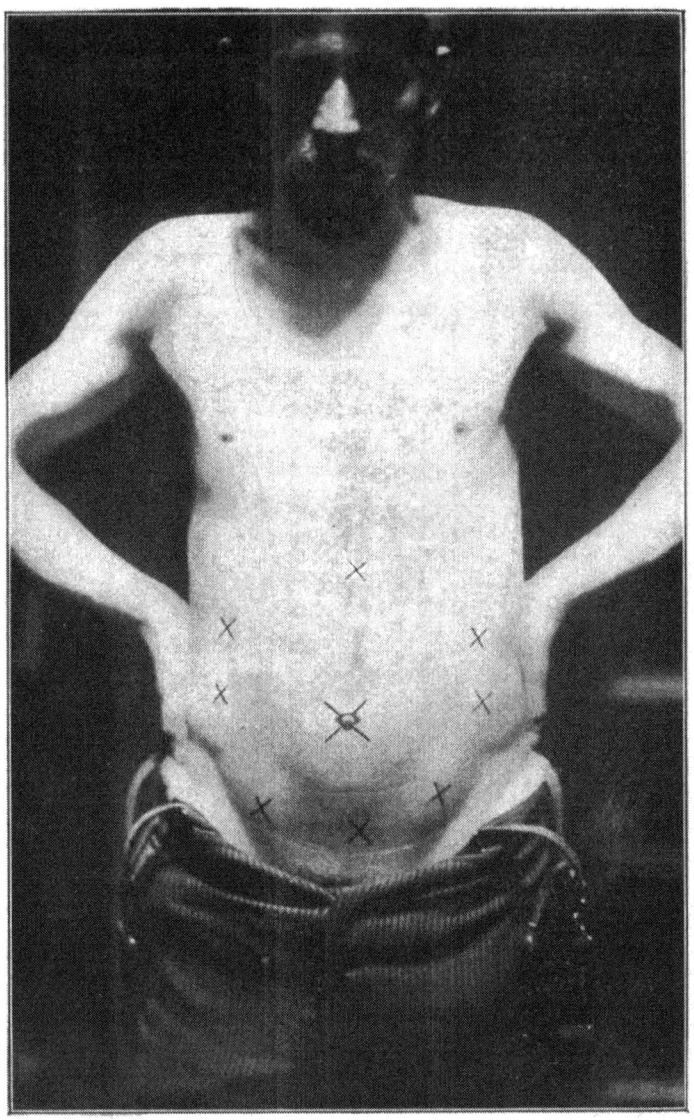

Fig. 1.—Points of election on the abdominal surface, marked by crosses, for executing auto-massage.

CHAPTER VIII.

THE TREATMENT OF SPLANCHNIC NEURASTHENIA.

THE FUNDAMENTAL PRINCIPLES GOVERNING TREATMENT. THE PHYSICAL METHODS OF TREATMENT; ABDOMINAL MASSAGE, ABDOMINAL EXERCISES, RESPIRATORY EXERCISES, ELECTRICITY, ABDOMINAL SUPPORTERS, AND HYDROTHERAPY. — CITATION OF CASES OF SPLANCHNIC NEURASTHENIA. — ACTION OF PURGATIVES IN SPLANCHNIC NEURASTHENIA.

THE primary and fundamental condition prevailing in splanchnic neurasthenia is a stagnation of blood in the splanchnic or abdominal veins. This condition is either primary or secondary to nervous exhaustion. The treatment then, must not only embrace the neurasthenic state, but the local condition of abdominal plethora. The general treatment of neurasthenia has already been discussed in Chapter V. This much is true, however: 1. That if neurasthenia is dependent on congestion of the intra-abdominal veins, any treatment directed toward the former, however effective, will only result in temporary benefit. 2. Treatment directed toward the relief of abdominal congestion alone will often permanently arrest the neurasthenic symptoms. 3. Practically all cases of neurasthenia are associated with abdominal congestion, which serves to aggravate the neurasthenic symptoms, insomuch as one of the earliest evidences of nerve waste is a diminished tone of the abdominal sympathetic. 4. There are many instances of abdominal congestion which never present the picture of neurasthenia, but are manifested by an ill-defined group of symptoms, which baffle classification under any recognized form of disease. In any case, the relief and cure of abdominal congestion is imperative. I give expression to a conservative statement when I say, that in no other form of neurasthenia are results achieved so positively, quickly, and permanently, as in the splanchnic form of the affection. Here, our therapeutic maneuvers cannot bear the imprint of suggestion, for we can control the results of treatment by certain objective signs which are indisputable, viz.: The reduction of hepatic enlargement, the disappearance of hepatic and abdominal tenderness, and the diminished grade of the Cardio-splanchnic phenomenon; and the gradual abatement of the objective signs run parallel with the evanescence of the subjective symptoms. We will now proceed to a discussion of the physical methods which are designed to correct congestion of the abdominal veins.

PHYSICAL METHODS WHICH CURE SPLANCHNIC NEURASTHENIA BY RELIEVING CONGESTION OF THE ABDOMINAL VEINS: 1. *Massage of the abdominal wall;* 2. *Exercises which strengthen the abdominal muscles;* 3. *Respiratory exercises;* 4. *Electricity to the abdomen;* 5. *Abdominal supporters;* 6. *Cold water.*

MASSAGE OF THE ABDOMINAL WALL. When reference is made to this maneuver, it does not signify the conventional massage, but a form of massage, executed by the patient, which achieves three distinct objects: 1. It strengthens the abdominal muscles which, by their

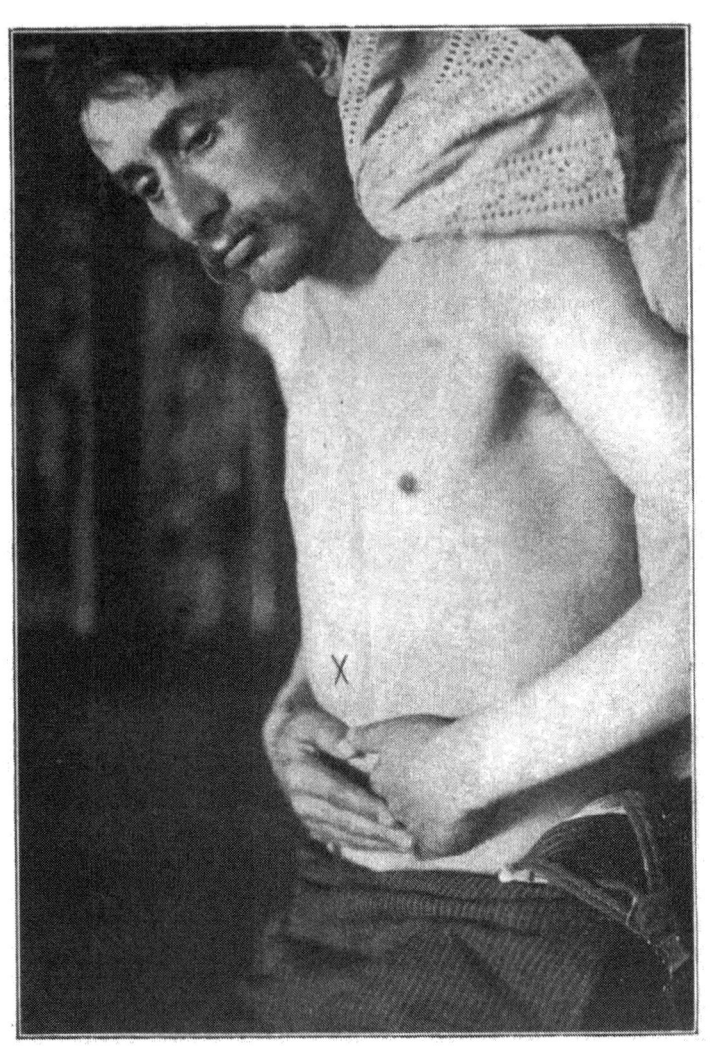

Fig. 2.—Method for executing auto-massage. The patient is in the recumbent posture with knees well drawn up so as to relax the muscles of the abdomen.

augmented tone, increase intra-abdominal tension, thus clamping the intra-abdominal veins, as it were, and preventing their engorgement; 2. It facilitates the return of blood from the abdominal veins to the heart; 3. It favorably influences reflexly the sympathetic nerve fibers which dominate the supply of blood to the abdominal organs.

METHOD OF ABDOMINAL MASSAGE. 1. Method of expulsion; 2. Respiratory method.

METHOD OF EXPULSION. This method is designed for the comparatively strong subject, for it must be remembered that abdominal manipulations of any kind act reflexly on the heart.* To aid in the elucidation of this maneuver, reference is made to the accompanying illustrations: In figure 1, the abdomen is marked by crosses, which indicate the points of election for executing abdominal massage. In figure 2, the fingers are in contact with one of these points. The fingers of the left hand are first placed on the abdominal wall with a varying degree of pressure, which is re-enforced by superimposed pressure with the fingers of the other hand. The subject next endeavors, by contraction of the abdominal muscles, to overcome the pressure exerted by the fingers. This constitutes the complete act of *automassage*. It is repeated ten or more times over each spot, depending on the endurance of the subject. When the spots contiguous to the curvature of the ribs are reached, the fingers must be passed as far as possible under the ribs. The subject executes massage in the recumbent posture, as this position best favors the return of blood to the heart. The legs as seen in the illustration are well drawn up to relax the abdominal muscles,

* Appendix, Note 8.

so that they may be more easily and powerfully contracted. The vigor of the massage may be gradually increased by increasing the pressure of the fingers and the
number of manipulations over each spot. Massage executed after the foregoing manner may be followed by a
sense of oppression in the heart region and fulness in
the head, sensations which may be referred to over-dis-
tension of the heart, due to the large quantities of blood
expressed into this organ from the abdominal veins.
After each contraction of the abdominal muscles, the
subject should take a *forced deep breath,* so as to suck
the blood into the lungs from the engorged right heart:
an act which will easily remove and prevent the sensations already referred to. The sensation of tingling,
which the patient experiences in the extremities during
massage, are rather pleasant than otherwise, and may
be referred to an improved circulation. Soreness of the
abdomen after initiation of the exercises may be disregarded, being provoked by contraction of muscles unaccustomed to exercise.

RESPIRATORY METHOD. This is a maneuver less
harsh than the former, having for its goal the same objects, and designed for subjects in whom the heart-action
is not strong. As in the expulsion method, the fingers
are placed in succession over each spot with a varying
degree of pressure and by a forced act of inspiration
only, the patient endeavors to remove the pressure exerted by the fingers. maneuver may be repeated
over each spot a varying number of times, and the finger
pressure increased or diminished, according to the endurance of the subject. There are certain facts worthy
of mention in reference to this form of auto-massage.
As a rule, splanchnic neurasthenics suffer from hemor-

rhoids, and this is not extraordinary, considering the engorgement of the abdominal veins. Auto-massage will cure such hemorrhoids, not only in neurasthenics, but in others, and I know of no simpler nor more effective measure for the relief and cure of this obstinate affection. In reference to auto-massage on the action of the bowels, all I can say is this, that some splanchnic neurasthenics obtain relief from their constipation, others find no relief, whereas others, who are not constipated, increase the number of their bowel movements. In any event auto-massage will do much toward augmenting the tone of the intestines.

EXERCISES WHICH STRENGTHEN THE ABDOMINAL MUSCLES. These exercises may be employed in conjunction with auto-massage, or either may be executed to the exclusion of the other, although if either method is employed alone, preference is given to auto-massage. Exercises for developing the abdominal muscles must be regulated in duration and number by the age and strength of the patient.

These exercises should be avoided if hernia exists, unless primarily supervised by the physician.

EXERCISE 1. Rope-hauling exercise. Two strong elastic cords, two feet in length and fixed into the floor at one end, while to the free end rings are attached which can be grasped by the hands. These cords are stretched alternately by first pulling with one and then with the other hand, as in rope-hauling.

EXERCISE 2. The patient lies on the floor and places his feet against some resisting object, and then attempts to assume the sitting posture. This exercise may be repeated a number of times. When the patient begins

the exercises, he may assist himself in rising by aid
of the hands.

EXERCISE 3. This requires the aid of an assistant.
The patient, seated on a stool, bends his body back-
wards and forwards. The forward movement is resisted
by the assistant, who grasps the shoulders from behind.

EXERCISE 4. The patient sits on a stool with his
back to the wall. On either side of him is a ring fixed
into the wall. Through each ring a cord passes, to the
ends of which weights are attached. The portion of
cord between the two rings is passed round the waist.
The body is then repeatedly bent toward the thighs and
the weights thereby raised. (Campbell.)

STRENGTHENING THE ABDOMINAL MUSCLES BY
MEANS OF AN EXERCISER. I have devised a simple apparatus (see illustrations, figs. 3 and 4), which I regard
as most serviceable in this connection. The work put
upon the abdominal muscles by means of this apparatus
can be regulated to any degree, depending on the amount
of traction put upon the elastic cords. It consists of 4
pieces of elastic cord, each one-half inch in width and
about 5 feet in length; a firm though yielding belt of
leather, very smooth on the surface, brought in contact
with the abdomen 4 inches in width and tapered at
the ends and provided with strap and buckle for fixation
around the abdomen; two blocks of wood, provided with
4 holes for the elastic cords, each piece five inches in
width and about an inch in thickness. To each block
of wood a piece of firm leather is screwed, leaving a
projecting loop, which, in appearance, is not unlike a
stirrup. The leather stirrups are intended for the at-
tachment of snaps. The elastic cords are fixed by means
of a knot in each hole in one block of wood, the cord in

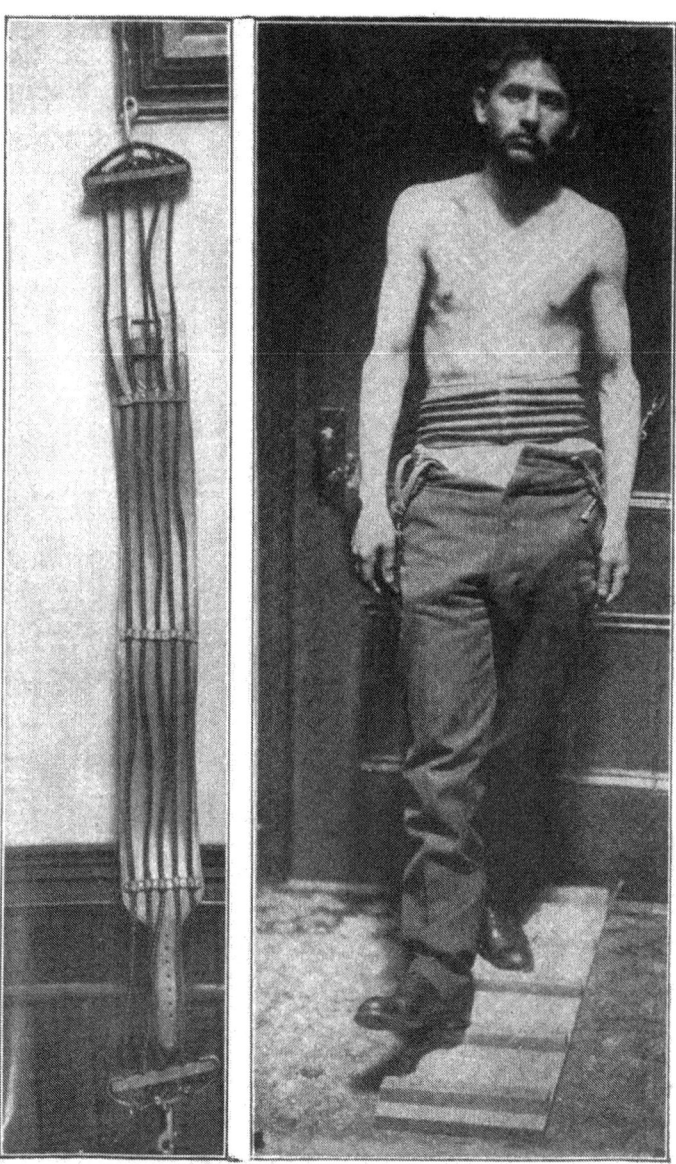

Fig. 3.—Apparatus for abdominal exercises.

Fig. 4.—Method of using the apparatus for abdominal exercises.

contact with the holes being wound with fine wire to prevent wear; then they pass across the front of the leather belt, and to prevent slipping, across the belt three narrow strips of leather, vertically attached by means of rivets, are placed, with apertures for the cords; then the cords are passed through the holes of the other block of wood, and fixed by means of knots, and here likewise re-enforced by wire. The apparatus is then attached to two screw eyes in the wall, when it is ready for use.

The elastic cords, shown in the illustration, are covered with webbing, and after a limited use of the apparatus, become worn, leaving the rubber free. This is a serious objection, and for this reason, solid rubber cords, two in number and about one inch in width may be employed; otherwise, the apparatus is made according to the description already given. It is a matter of little moment what kind of apparatus is employed, provided it permits of regulated abdominal traction.

The belt of the apparatus is first placed below the navel and tightened by means of the strap and buckle; then the patient steps forward on a board placed on the floor, which is provided with cleats arranged at convenient distances. The real work is executed while stepping forward, the backward movement being effected by the elasticity of the cords. The number of tractions made by the abdomen is regulated by the strength and endurance of the patient. After the lower abdomen is exercised, the belt is fixed successively on the navel, and then above the navel, so that all parts of the abdominal muscles may be included in the exercises. I advise my patients that, after each traction by means of the abdomen, a *deep inspiration* should be taken to prevent

accumulation of blood in the heart and to further its
circulation through the body. I further advise my
patients to exercise after rising and before retiring; to
begin with 10 tractions, in each position of the belt, viz.:
below, at and above the navel, 30 in all; and to gradually increase the number to 75.

RESPIRATORY EXERCISES. We have already referred
in a previous chapter to the great value of *pulmonary
ventilation,* in preventing disease and maintaining the
standard of health. The lungs are important avenues
for the elimination of poisonous substances generated
within the body; they regulate the local and general
blood and lymph circulations, not only in a quantitative, but in a qualitative manner. Without properly developed lungs, no individual can be regarded as healthy.
While general exercises may and do contribute to respiratory gymnastics, the character of the exercises is
such that it is more than the average patient can do,
hence local *pulmonary gymnastics* are necessary for the
preservation of health. We have already shown that the
mere act of inspiration performs a double function in
relieving abdominal congestion, viz.: The descent of the
diaphragm, by increasing intra-abdominal tension,
squeezes the blood out of the intra-abdominal veins into
the heart; inspiration favors pulmonary suction, for
during this phase of respiration, the blood-vessels of the
lungs are expanded, and the blood is sucked, not only
out of the abdominal veins, but from the veins throughout the body. It is only rarely in health that the lungs
in their entirety are physiologically active, and this
question is further discussed in the appendix.* Both
phases of respiration may be influenced by respiratory

* Appendix, Note 1.

gymnastics, viz.: inspiration and expiration or both. In the average case, it may be presumed that when inspiration is vigorous, expiration is equally vigorous, but in those predisposed to pulmonary tuberculosis, we may have, as my investigations show, a voluminous lung capable of performing the act of inspiration with normal vigor, and yet the expiratory act may be seriously compromised.* Here attention will be directed to a simple exercise for facilitating inspiration, and it may be executed in conjunction with the use of the abdominal apparatus previously described. I believe I am justified in protesting against prolix methods for securing lung development. Such methods accomplish little and defeat their object, which cause them soon to be relinquished. The Roentgen rays have furnished me with indisputable proof in selecting simple methods for inflating the lungs.

It is well known that the lungs in health appear in the fluoroscopic picture as light areas. The lungs appear brighter during inspiration than expiration; in fact, the greater the lung inflation, the brighter the reflex. I have examined patients with the fluoroscope during the time "breathing tubes" were used, and while the different postures and exercises were practiced, as advocated by various writers, and I was unable to demonstrate that any method was superior to that of forced breathing. In fact, in some of the advocated methods, the fluoroscope demonstrated the lung phase to be really that of expiration, whereas, the object supposed to be attained was lung inflation. To enhance the value of forced inspiration with the object of attaining hyperventilation of the lungs, the simple expedient of holding

* Appendix, Note 7.

the breath after full inspiration will be found of great value. After a little practice, patients are able to hold the breath fully two minutes. If, during this maneuver, regional percussion is made, it will be found that the position of the lung borders extend beyond the limits attained by forced inspiration alone. The principle involved in explanation of the foregoing phenomenon is one relating to pneumatics, by raising the temperature of a gas we increase the volume. Another simple maneuver is to direct the patient, after taking a forced inspiration, to count slowly. With a little practice, 80 can be counted without difficulty. This is an exercise both for the inspiratory and expiratory forces. For rapid lung development, inhalations of compressed air by the aid of the pneumatic cabinet, is unquestionably the best method. After a limited course of treatment the thoracic capacity may be increased 2 per cent., with a corresponding development both of chest measurements and chest expansion.

The method which I earnestly advocate, when used in connection with the abdominal exerciser, is that employed by the Swedish trainers, and after each or several tractions are made by the abdomen, this exercise is executed. It is as follows: The patient raises his arms to the vertical position, at the same time taking a deep inspiration. He then brings the arms downward and backward, thus describing a large movement of circumduction. When the patient practices forced inspiration, he supports himself on his toes, inclining his body backward during the entire period of inspiration.

ELECTRICITY TO THE ABDOMEN.* Of all methods, this is unquestionably the most expeditious and thor-

* Appendix, Note 13.

ough in the treatment of splanchnic neurasthenia, and were I less conservative, I would regard it as a specific measure. I have tested all forms of electricity, physiologically and therapeutically, in relation to this special affection, viz.: Galvanic, faradic, static and high frequency, but they are all subservient in their action to the Sinusoidal Current.

The *Sinusoidal Current* * acts differently upon the body from other forms of current, and this is due to the number of alternations in a second, the quantity of current, and the degree of electro-motive force. Owing to the uniformity of the alternations, *strong currents may be employed* without producing pain or muscular contractions. The sinusoidal current possesses the property of contracting the organs, specially the heart, inducing what I have called the *heart reflex,* the lungs (*lung reflex of contraction*) and the liver (*liver reflex*).† It is also endowed with the property of contracting the veins, notable the intra-abdominal veins and of stimulating the sympathetic abdominal nerve fibers.

The effect of this current in driving the blood from the intra-abdominal veins back into the heart is evidenced by the cardio-splanchnic phenomenon, which is elicited to a remarkable degree after its application. The sinusoidal current, by the uniformity of its alternations, anesthetizes the terminal sympathetic nerve fibers and this anesthesia is so marked in the skin between the electrodes that no sensation is experienced by the patient, even after a pin prick during the application of the current.

My usual method of application is to place one large

* Appendix, Note 6.
† Appendix, Note 18.

electrode above and another below the navel and fix them in position by means of straps. The duration of each application made daily must not be less than 15 minutes. Not infrequently while one electrode is applied to the abdomen the other may be applied to the back of the neck, specially if the patient complains of pains radiating to the back of the neck. Each application is, as a rule, followed by a sensation of well-being, which is never attained so expeditiously by any other method of treatment. The strength of the current should be as strong as the patient can tolerate, but never too strong to induce unpleasant sensations.

I have also employed *vibratory massage of the abdomen* by means of a vibratory machine, as a substitute for the sinusoidal current, but the effects can in no wise be compared to the current.

ABDOMINAL SUPPORTERS. The use of a properly-fitting abdominal support or belt is only to be thought of when the abdominal muscles are relaxed beyond the hope of restoration by electricity, exercise, massage, etc. There can be no objection, however, to use a support in connection with the methods already referred to for strengthening the abdominal muscles. The physician should examine the support to determine whether it merits its name, insomuch as the majority of abdominal supporters on the market are worse than useless. In dislocation of the abdominal viscera (*Enteroptosis*) the wearing of an abdominal supporter affords much relief to the wearer. The relief thus attained is not due wholly to reposition of the organs, as is instanced in the observations of Bial.[35] The latter applied transparent bandages to cases of gastroptosis and transilluminated the stomachs before and after the application of the bandages. No change in the position of the stomach could be noted, and it is therefore most likely that abdominal supporters act chiefly by compression of the viscera, which in turn squeeze the blood out of the turgid abdominal veins.

COLD WATER. After the morning exercises with the abdominal apparatus, I insist on my patients taking a lukewarm bath, or even a cold bath, if they are accustomed to it, and by means of a spray douche direct cold water from a certain height to fall on different parts of the abdomen. This is a most effective means of augmenting the tone of the abdominal walls, and organs and tissues of the abdomen. The circulation of the blood, the motion of the alimentary canal and the process of nutrition are thus stimulated reflexly by innumerable nerves which terminate in the skin.

In concluding the subject of treatment for splanchnic neurasthenia, it may be mentioned for the sake of completeness, that, when the anterior abdominal wall is beyond hope of repair, owing to its flabby and relaxed condition, an operation may be suggested for its resection. This operation has been performed with success by different surgeons. I have selected ten cases among my splanchnic neurasthenics to illustrate the effects of treatment according to the lines already laid down.

CASE I. *Vertiginous Symptoms.* Merchant. Age 42. Pronounced symptoms of neurasthenia. The chief symptom is vertigo, which has increased of late to such a degree that he fears to go out without a companion. One evening he had eaten too heartily of fresh fruit, with the result that he developed an attack of intestinal colic, and his vertigo became very much intensified. He noted with much surprise that the pressure of his wife's hands on his abdomen, while relieving his symptoms of colic, likewise gave temporary relief to his vertigo. His wife suggested the application of a bandage to his abdomen, with the result that as long as the bandage was worn, the vertigo disappeared. After recovery from his colic, he was able to go about unattended, provided he wore a closely-fitting leather belt around his abdomen, and if this belt were removed, the signs of vertigo would recur. This case suggested to me the pertinent fact, that the patient in question owed his vertiginous attacks to gravitation of blood to the splanchnic area, and that the application of his leather belt merely forced the blood from the latter area into the general circulation. After one month's treatment by means of the sinusoidal current, daily applications, supplemented by abdominal and respiratory exercises, the patient dispensed with his leather belt, and was, in fact, cured. In this and other cases, it is difficult to say how permanent the cure really is, and for this reason, I enjoin my patients to continue their exercises for an indefinite period.

CASE II.   Chief symptom, *pain* radiating to the arms and legs. Tailor; age 38. Has been unable to follow his occupation for the last eight months, owing to paroxysms of pain, which radiate to the neck, arms and legs. His arms feel " like paralyzed," and legs seem unable to support his body. Has headaches. Suffers from gas in the stomach and bowels. Has been losing in weight, and cannot sleep. Has been subjected to almost all kinds of treatment by different physicians, without any relief. Examination shows an enlarged and sensitive liver, in fact, palpation of this organ almost " causes him to faint." His abdominal wall lacks tone.

Treatment by means of the sinusoidal current, one electrode to the back of the neck and the other to the abdomen, supplemented by exercises, has enabled him, after five weeks treatment, to return to work.

CASE III. *Mental symptoms.* Clerk; aged 29. Has had syphilis. Has a feeling of pressure on the top of his head. He is in constant dread that "something is going to happen." Feels as though something were lodged in his "belly," and that by taking a deep breath he is able temporarily to dislodge it. While in my presence during his early visits to my office, he was constantly engaged in taking forced inspirations. His memory is poor, and he is unable to concentrate his attention on anything. Examination demonstrated the conventional stigmata of splanchnic neurasthenia. This patient had taken three rest cures and for more than a year had traveled about the country in search of health. After two months' treatment, he was able to resume his work, when he said "I never felt better in my life."

CASE IV. Chief symptoms, *depression* and *weakness.* Woman; married; age 46. Could not be persuaded to leave her bed on account of extreme weakness. Was very much depressed, and feared that her relatives were going to take her to an insane asylum. She eats only sparingly, contending that food distresses her. Her history prior to her illness, which has been gradual in its approach, was uneventful. Examination showed no liver enlargement nor tenderness. There was only one point of abdominal tenderness. Pressure on the abdomen, kept up for several minutes, demonstrated the cardio-splanchnic phenomenon to an unusual degree. Treatment was begun with the sinusoidal current to the abdomen, and after two weeks, she could be persuaded to take the other exercises, with the result that in three months she was discharged as cured.

CASE V. Prominent symptom, *pain in the liver region.* Woman; married; age 43. Is very much depressed on account of pains in the region of the liver. "Bloats" after eating. Has symptoms of indigestion. Is constipated. Liver enlarged and tender. Abdominal points of tenderness. After two weeks treatment patient returned home and, as she said, "completely cured."

CASE VI. Prominent symptom, "*the blues.*" Electrician; age 40. Has no symptoms beyond attacks of "the blues." Knows no cause for their occurrence. The attacks may last a week, during which period he is unfit for his occupation. Examination reveals the stigmata of splanchnic neurasthenia. Self-treatment by massage and exercises. The result of treatment has been that his blues, as he says, "are now a matter of history only."

CASE VII. Chief symptom, *impotency.* Teacher; age 31; married. Very nervous and irritable. Always depressed. Worries about his sexual condition. Has attempted suicide. Associates his impotency with intestinal indigestion, insomuch as he finds that whenever he belches much gas, his sexual condition is worse. Stigmata of splanchnic neurasthenia. Self-treatment by massage practiced twice daily. After the third treatment, improvement became manifest, and after four weeks, he asserted that his sexual power was restored.

CASE VIII. Prominent symptom, *palpitation of the heart.* Banker; married; age 53. Suffered for years from palpitation of the heart. Attacks have become more frequent and of longer duration. Worse after eating. Cardiac palpitation is associated with symptoms of indigestion. Fears that he has heart disease. Has consulted many prominent physicians in this country and Europe. Has submitted to all kinds of treatment, including a rest cure, lasting three months. Liver not enlarged. No signs of organic heart disease. No abdominal points of tenderness. Pulse rate, 90 per minute, and can be reduced to normal after repeated pressure on the abdomen. Treatment by means of the sinusoidal current, and cure after three weeks treatment. It may be remarked incidentally, that in this patient, there were no stigmata of splanchnic neurasthenia, beyond the *exaggerated presence* of the *cardio-splanchnic phenomenon,* and this is the only clue to the affection in a number of cases.

CASE IX. Prominent symptom, *indigestion.* Capitalist; aged 62. Very much depressed and generally nervous. Has a constant burning in the stomach. Does not eat much on account of the food, which distresses him. Has lost 25 pounds in weight. Nothing relieves him. Has a pendulous abdomen. The stomach is dilated and dislocated. The liver is very much enlarged, and is very sensitive to pressure. Abdominal points of tenderness. Treatment, sinusoidal current to the abdomen and auto-massage. Relief after one week and cure in seven weeks.

CASE X. Prominent symptom, *morbid fears.* Woman; aged 28. Fears crowds and open spaces. Will not handle door knobs, fearing infection. Very irritable and "blue." Symptoms of indigestion. Faints easily. Has headaches, and is *constipated.* Purgatives intensify her symptoms, therefore, she allows herself to remain constipated rather than take a purgative. Exami-

nation reveals all the characteristic symptoms of splanchnic neurasthenia. Treatment by auto-massage resulted
in cure.

ACTION OF PURGATIVES IN SPLANCHNIC NEURAS-
THENIA. The recital of the last case directs our attention to the use of purgatives in this particular affection.
As a rule, physicians, presuming that these cases respond
in their symptomatic make-up to intestinal auto-toxemia,
have habitual recourse to intestinal antiseptics and cathartics. Now, cathartics in such subjects, in my experience, act unfavorably, for they induce a feeling of
faintness or vertigo and intensify the nervous symptoms.
The reason for all this is evident. Cathartics induce, by
their action, the determination of an increased supply
of blood to the abdominal organs, thereby augmenting
the symptoms dependent on congestion of the intra-abdominal veins. I know several individuals who are constrained to defecate in the recumbent posture, otherwise they will suffer from faintness. The faintness experienced by persons when they first assume the vertical
posture after a prolonged illness owes its genesis to the
same cause which operates in the instances already
mentioned. Hill and Barnard [36] have shown the influence of gravity on the circulation and the part performed by the abdominal muscles in preventing the
gravitation of blood into the splanchnic veins. They
demonstrated that when the splanchnic vasomotor mechanism was intact, it was able to prevent such gravitation,
but when this mechanism was destroyed by section of the
splanchnic nerves, a second mechanism was brought into
operation, consisting of expiratory compressions of the
abdomen, occurring simultaneously with inspiratory
thoracic suctions, the former squeezing, the latter suck-

ing the blood out of the splanchnic pool. Now faintness occurring when the vertical posture is assumed, means any one of three things, viz.: Diminished intraabdominal tension from relaxed abdominal walls, diminished thoracic suction or an enfeebled state of the splanchnic vasomotor system. The loss of one mechanism may and often is compensated by another.

The mechanism consisting of abdominal compressions in expiration and thoracic suctions in inspirations, as well as the splanchnic vasomotor mechanism, may be destroyed by division of the cord at the first dorsal vertebra. If the animal operated on be then held vertically with the head up, all the blood will collect in the splanchnic veins, and the empty heart continues vainly to beat; but after compressing the abdomen, the blood is squeezed into the heart, thus restoring the circulation.

APPENDIX.

THE physiologic principles involved in respiration are
not always strictly in accord with clinical observation.
By this I mean that civilized man has so subverted
primeval respiration, by attire and modes of living, that
what is now regarded as physiologic, is really pathologic. Physiology teaches that the lungs, even at the
termination of expiration, are in a stretched condition,
and the experiment is frequently cited of making an
opening into the pleural cavity, which drives a certain
amount of air into the trachea. Without entering further into a discussion of this matter, let us learn to what
degree such physiologic teaching is in conflict with clinical evidence. The lungs do not by any means fully
occupy the thoracic space. The costal and visceral lay-
ers of the pleura make up a sac in which, so to speak,
the lungs are let in. In certain thoracic situations the
pleural sac is larger than the lung volume, and forms
spaces, known as *pleural* or *reserve spaces*. Such spaces
permit of changes in the lung volume, which otherwise
would be impossible. The pleural spaces exist throughout the entire extent of the lung borders, the largest,
known as the sinus phrenicocostalis, being located at the
lower outer lung-border, at a point where the costal
passes over into the diaphragmatic pleura. Figs. 5

and 6 show the sites of the pleural spaces (shaded) on the anterior and lateral aspects of the thorax.

Even the deepest inspirations are not sufficient to cause the lungs to fully occupy the pleural spaces. The pleural space on the lateral aspect of the thorax may be filled, if the patient lies on the opposite side and conducts deep and forced inspirations. In quiet respiration, the difference in the position of the lower lung-borders during the respiratory phase is about 1 cm.,

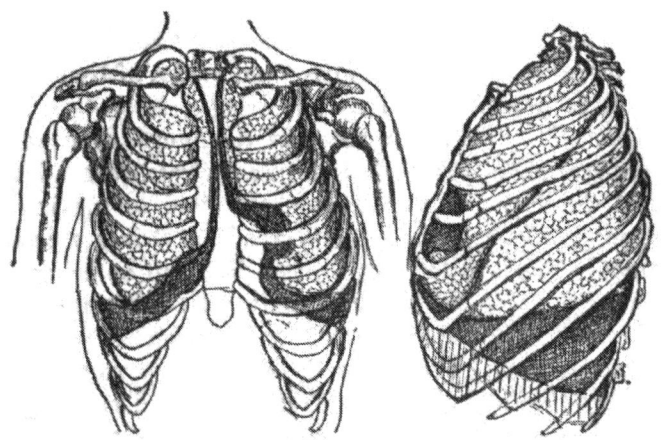

Fig. 5. Showing pleural spaces shaded. (Eichhorst), Fig. 6. Pleural spaces (shaded) on the lateral surface of the left lung. (Eichhorst.)

whereas, if the respiratory excursions are more pronounced, especially in the lateral chest region, the difference may be as great as 13 cm. This active mobility of the lung borders is always greater than the passive mobility, which is influenced by the body posture. Having succinctly reviewed these anatomic facts, we will now present the clinical findings, which contravene the

* *American Medicine*, Feb. 15, 1902.

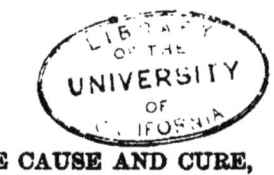

assumption of the physiologist, that the lungs are always in a stretched condition. I have frequently directed attention in the literature to constant areas of diminished lung resonance, varying from dulness to flatness, as obtained by percussion. In number and situation these areas vary, but they admit in the aggregate of definite localization. These areas of dulness, or *atelectatic zones,* as I have called them, possess one characteristic feature, they may be dispelled by repeated forced inspirations. By this simple maneuver, resonance will supplant dulness. The atelectatic zones are dependent

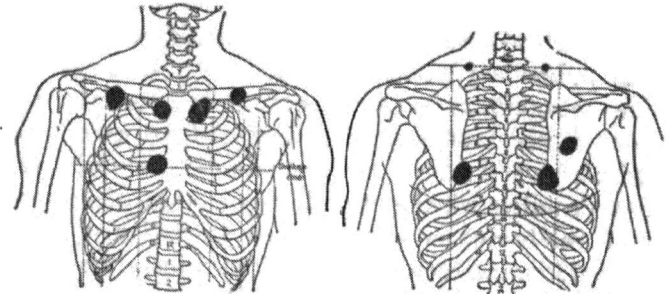

Fig. 7.—Patches on the front surface of chest.　　Fig 8.—Patches on the posterior surface of chest.

on circumscribed pulmonary atelectasis or collapse of limited portions of the lung, and dissociated with any demonstrable lesion. While it is true from the standpoint of the physiologist, that the lungs are in a stretched condition, it is equally true from the position of the clinician that certain portions of the lungs are collapsed and deprived of sufficient air to yield a dulness, and in some instances, a flatness on percussion. The atelectatic zones vary in size from a 25-cent piece to a dollar, or even larger, and are permanently absent when the lungs are emphysematous, and temporarily so, after repeated deep inspirations, but they reappear in a few minutes, when tranquil breathing is resumed. In Figs. 7 and 8 I have projected a composite picture defining the situation of the atelectatic zones, based on an examination of over 100 apparently healthy persons, children as well as adults. On the posterior surface of the chest, the zones are more frequently encountered, and admit of more definite localization than those on the anterior surface of the thoracic wall. Since the advent of the Röntgen rays, I have observed the following: (1) Atelectatic zones throw circumscribed shadows on the fluoroscope, which will vary according to the degree and area of the pulmonary atelectasis. (2) The shadows cast by the atelectatic zones can be made to disappear by continuous forced breathing, and they will reappear after a variable period when quiet breathing is resumed. (3) Before deciding whether the shadow cast on the fluoroscope is really due to pulmonary consolidation, the subject should be instructed to make forced inspirations; if the shadow disappears, and is supplanted by a bright reflex, it is due to atelectasis; if the shadow persists, pulmonary consolidation may safely be concluded to exist, excluding, of course, other anatomic conditions that would interfere with the transmission of the Röntgen rays to the fluoroscope. (4) Skiascopy of the lungs demonstrates that the opacities on the fluoroscope, corresponding to the atelectatic zones, greatly exceed the percussional areas of the latter, and, furthermore, that in individuals in whom no zones can be demonstrated by percussion, opacities are sometimes present, which disappear after forced inspiration. (5) Before and during a radioscopic examination of the lungs it is always imperative to instruct the patient to practice forced breathing.

What are the practical conclusions that may be formulated as a result of the foregoing observations? Danger may accrue from confounding the physical signs of atelectatic dulness with dulness caused by lung consolidation, an error which can always be avoided, if the patient is directed to practice forced inspirations before percussion of the chest is attempted. Whenever a localized dulness of the lung is detected, it is a wise provision to instruct the patient to take a series of deep breaths; if the dulness disappears, we are dealing with an atelectatic zone, if, however, the dulness persists, we are justified in concluding that there is some lung anomaly. I hold that topographic percussion, as obtained ordinarily, is of inconstant value. The limitation of organs by percussion, especially the heart, will vary from day to day, and the percussional area of dulness in the same case and at the same time will be variously obtained by different diagnosticians. The borders of the liver, heart, and spleen are dependent on the degree of the lung inflation, and must vary according to the activity of respiration. Topographic percussion must always be based on the state of pulmonary inflation, and the results governed accordingly. The aid afforded by auscultation in the elimination of atelectasis is obvious. Auscultation of the lungs should be conducted with the patient in different postures, the object being to utilize the actual respiratory capacity of the lungs, thus eliminating the auscultatory phenomena of atelectasis and accentuating abnormal sounds, which may be present. The recognition of the atelectatic zones is of the greatest

importance to the skiascopist, as failure to recognize
them may lead to the grave error of misinterpreting the
shadows cast on the fluoroscope as evidence of lung
tuberculosis. Stubbert, in a contribution, maintains
that he is unable to confirm my observations relative to
the atelectatic zones. It is gratifying, however, for me
to add, that Cabot, in his recent book, makes mention
of my observations, and confirms them. Any physician
who places sole reliance on percussion, or the shadows
cast on the fluoroscope, as evidence of lung consolidation, will commit the
egregious blunder of
interpreting tuber-
culosis in more than
50 per cent. of the
patients coming to
him for examination.

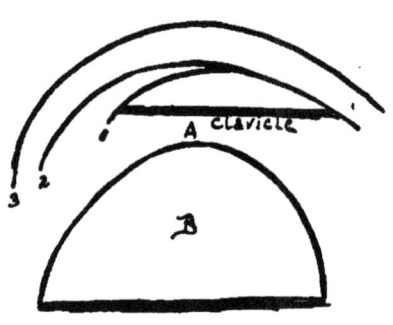

In Fig. 9 A. we
observe the fluoros-
cope reproduction of
the lung apex in a
normal individual.
Note the area

Fig. 9.—*A, c,* Clavicle. 1. Area of apex in normal breathing. 2. Apical
area in deep breathing. 3 Apical area after elicitation of lung reflex. *B,*
Apical area after strapping the lower chest.

of luminosity represented by the apex in tranquil breathing. (1) Observe how this area is augmented after
forced deep breathing (2) and again after elicitation
of the lung reflex (3). Observe the extraordinary increase in luminosity after strapping the lower chest
which permits of breathing in the upper chest only (B).
A word of caution is necessary to those who are desirous

of confirming the latter observations. Owing to the
extraordinary respiration in the upper chest area, the
clavicles may obscure by their elevation, the luminous
apical area, hence, the latter area should only be gauged
when the patient practices forced expiration, which will
cause a descent of the clavicles.

I have already mentioned the fact that the atelectatic
zones may be dissipated by forced inspirations, but this
is not always true, for there are instances when only
repeated forced inhalations of compressed air will cause
their evanescence. There are two methods, which will
cause their disappearance: by evoking the lung reflex,*
which will be referred to later, and by change in the
posture of the patient. The latter method I have only
observed recently. I found that, when the patient bends
forward for a few seconds, the zones can no longer be
elicited. This phenomenon I attribute to interference
with the movements of the diaphragm, which evokes
compensatory costal breathing. Not infrequently the
lung apex in its entirety is atelectatic and this may even
occur in a condition of apparent health. Kernig confirms this observation, to which I have frequently referred. Experience has taught me to regard most highly
the observation originally referred to by Seitz, the value
of percussing the upper borders of the lung apices, for
the earliest evidence of tuberculosis. Both apices rise
usually to the same height as determined by percussion, and the latter sign shows that the apices rise during inspiration and fall during expiration. Any difference in the height of the apices or any retarded dislocation during the phases of respiration must always be
regarded with grave suspicion. Figs. 10 and 11 show the

* Appendix, Note, 9.

normal height of the apices. Owing to the difficulty experienced in the exact demarcation of the apices anteriorly, I rely almost wholly on the evidence furnished on the posterior surface of the chest.

Atelectasis bears an important relation to *pulmonary tuberculosis* and *pulmonary anemia.* In the former affection, the zones bear an almost definite relation to the points of election and paths of distribution of the lesions in chronic pulmonary tuberculosis.

PULMONARY ANEMIA. In children, less often in

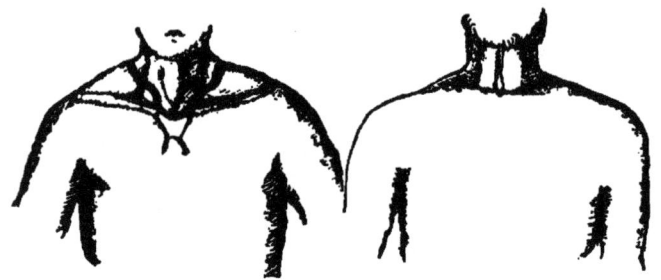

Fig. 10.—Extreme area of apical resonance on anterior surface of the chest.   Fig. 11.—Extreme area of apical resonance on the posterior surface of the chest.

adults, an anemia is often associated with atelectatic zones. This anemia I have designated as pulmonary. Pulmonary anemia attends multiplication or augmentation in area of the zones. The syndrome of anemia disappears upon a course of methodic respiratory gymnastics, while its recrudescence is always associated with a reappearance of the atelectatic zones. Pulmonary anemia is not an invariable concomitant of lung atelectasis, although as a rule, when anemia of pulmonary origin is present, atelectatic zones may be demonstrated.

In association with the anemia, fatigue on exertion, dyspnea, and heart palpitation, anomalies of digestion and constipation are usually present. Loss in weight is quite characteristic of pulmonary anemia, whereas, in the essential anemias, the well-nourished condition of the patient is manifest. There is another sign which distinguishes pulmonary from other forms of anemia, the one exception being, perhaps, progressive pernicious anemia, and that is, that while the ferruginous preparation benefit pure anemics, in pulmonary anemia they are practically valueless, at any rate, the benefit accruing from their use is evanescent. The real pathognomonic sign of pulmonary anemia is the therapeutic test. Subject such an individual to a single pneumatic cabinet treatment, employing inhalations of compressed air, and one invariably finds an increase in hemoglobin percentage if the anemia is of pulmonary genesis. The qnantity of iron in pulmonary anemia is probably normal, the element lacking is oxygen, and this hypothesis is evidently correct, inasmuch as all pulmonary anemics were cured by breathing exercises only. The recognition of pulmonary anemia as one of the earliest trustworthy signs of tuberculosis is of the greatest importance. I cannot adduce statistics in support of my contention, for that is a difficult matter. When, in the 18 years of my practice, I encountered an instance of pulmonary anemia, the patient was treated and not subjected to scientific observation, so it is impossible for me to say how many of my untreated cases of pulmonary anemia would have terminated in bacillary tuberculosis. There are certain observations in medicine which must be purely empiric. I will instance a few observations which have some bearing on this subject:

OBSERVATION I. In a tuberculous family, of whom three members died of the disease, two daughters came to my office for examination. In one daughter atelectatic zones were variously distributed over the chest.. Hemoglobin reduced to 60 per cent. Usual subjective symptoms of anemia. Treatment with the pneumatic cabinet. A period of five years has elapsed and the patient is still healthy. The other daughter also had the subjective symptoms of anemia, and the hemoglobin was reduced to 70 per cent. Only one atelectatic zone was present, situated on the anterior surface of the chest close to the manubrium sterni on the left side, and about three inches in circumference. This patient underwent no treatment. Two years later she returned to my office with pronounced tuberculosis. Cavitation of the lung corresponding to the atelectatic zone previously mentioned was evident. Six months later the patient died.

OBSERVATION II. A young man, aged 16. Pronounced evidence of anemia. Atelectatic zones present. Treatment with the pneumatic cabinet of short duration. Three years later the patient died of tuberculosis.

OBSERVATION III. Girl, aged 14. Hemoglobin reduced to 50 per cent. Red corpuscles reduced to 70 per cent. Atelectatic zones present. No other symptoms. One year later patient presented herself with symptoms of pulmonary tuberculosis. Patient cured.

The foregoing observations have been selected from a small number of analogous cases, and only justify the importance I have attached to pulmonary anemia as an early sign of tuberculosis. If pulmonary anemia is dependent on lung atelectasis, as I have attempted to show, the treatment indicated is lung development. All

my patients showed immediate and permanent improvement after daily inhalations of compressed air. The
color of the patients improved, the oxyhemoglobin and
number of red corpuscles increased and the subjective
signs of anemia disappeared. Whenever the organism
is compelled to dispose of more oxygen it produces more
oxygen carriers. If relapses occur, which were not infrequent, they were attributed in the main to neglect
of lung gymnastics or a return to former modes of life.

NOTE 2.—THE CARDIO-SPLANCHNIC PHENOMENON.*

MANY of the facts here recorded with reference to this phenomenon have appeared elsewhere in this work, but their importance will bear repetition.

To my knowledge this is an heretofore undescribed phenomenon, as far as its clinical manifestation is concerned. The facts, however, up to the point of its clinical identification have been fully established by the physiologic investigations of others. These facts are identified with intra-abdominal tension, and the effects of such tension on the blood circulation. Before describing the phenomenon in question, it will be apposite to succinctly review a few essential points on the subject of intra-abdominal tension. The latter in the norm is greater than the pressure of the atmosphere, and its positive pressure is exerted on the viscera which in turn press on the abdominal parietes, causing them to bulge. Should a reverse condition of things prevail, the walls of the abdomen would become retracted. Positive intra-abdominal pressure is subject to two conditions, viz.: the atmosphere pressure upon the yielding abdominal walls and the vigor of contraction of the abdominal muscles. For this reason, intra-abdominal pressure is

* American Journal of the Medical Sciences.

most pronounced in individuals with powerful muscles, and least evident in multiparous women with flaccid abdominal walls. Clinicians recognize the secondary effects of low intra-abdominal tension in conducing to splanchnoptosis, for, when the abdominal walls are relaxed as a permanent condition, their pressure on the underlying structures is insufficient, and the result is a ptosis of the viscera. The effects of reduced intra-abdominal tension on the circulation has received but scant consideration from clinicians, a most lamentable fact, considering the gravity of the issue involved. Hill and Barnard have largely contributed to this important subject, which has been practically elaborated in the excellent work of Campbell. They have demonstrated that there is a tendency of the blood to accumulate in the splanchnic area, with consequent syncope. Like the generality of veins, the great splanchnic veins are very susceptible to pressure, and the amount of blood within them is greatly influenced by the pressure of the abdominal walls. Mere pressure of the abdominal walls suffices to squeeze out of them a large quantity of blood. Thus gravity, posture, the accoutrements of dress, and other factors greatly influence the amount of blood contained in the splanchnic area. More blood accumulates in the splanchnic veins in the erect than in the recumbent posture, and it is not an uncommon observation for syncope to occur in bedridden patients who are suddenly constrained to get out of bed. The removal of stays in women often induces a feeling of faintness, and the same symptom may occur when a large quantity of ascitic fluid is removed and in susceptible subjects when the bladder is emptied or feces discharged. This feeling of faintness or syncope, while present in the normal

subject in the foregoing conditions, is greatly accentu-
ated when the abdominal walls are flaccid. Three factors
enter into consideration in the mechanism of blood supply to the splanchnic vessels, viz.: 1. The contraction
of the abdominal muscles; 2. The act of respiration, and,
3. The regulating vasomotor action of the splanchnic
vessels. The first factor is an important one, the transversales maintaining the anterior and posterior abdominal walls in fairly close contact and prevent in the erect
posture the gravitation of blood in the splanchnic area.
The second factor concerns the descent of the diaphragm
and pulmonary suction. Every time the diaphragm descends, the intra-abdominal vessels are compressed, and
the action thus exerted is less evident in the tense arteries
than in the flaccid veins: the blood being squeezed out
of the latter into the right heart. De Jager has shown
that even strong pressure upon the abdomen has little
or no effect on the arteries, but serves to squeeze a large
quantity of blood from the splanchnic veins. Hill has
also shown that, in consequence of some failure in certain compensatory mechanisms, the blood gravitates into
the splanchnic veins from the right heart, and that pressure upon the abdomen will send back the blood from
these veins to the right heart, and thus re-establish the
circulation. Such compression of the abdomen not only
augments the input into the right heart, but it likewise
increases, according to most writers, the systemic arterial pressure by increasing the peripheral resistance in
the splanchnic area.

Pulmonary suction refers to the large quantity of
blood drawn into the lungs with each inspiration, and
this physiologic process has not been inaptly compared
to a species of dry cupping. Chapman avers " that if, at

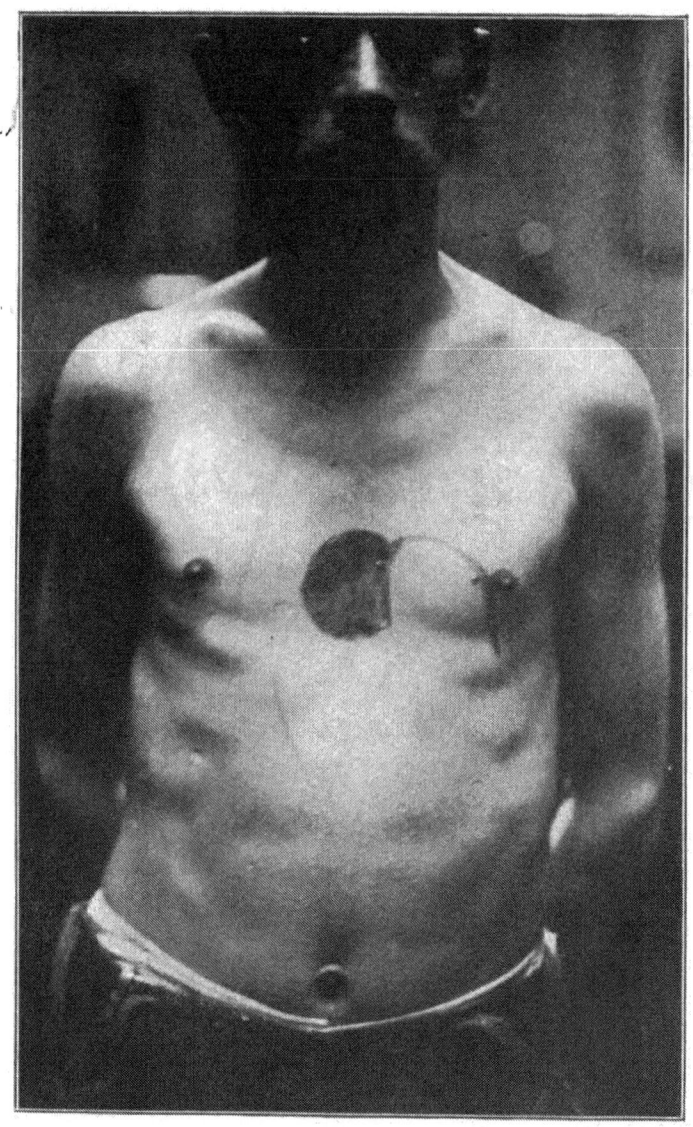

Fig. 12.—Illustrating the cardio-splanchnic phenomenon. The shaded area indicates the dull area obtained after vigorous compression of the abdomen. The contiguous area is the superficial area of cardiac dullness.

the termination of expiration, the quantity of blood in the lungs is from 1-15 to 1-18 of the total quantity of blood in the body, at the termination of inspiration, it will be from 1-12 to 1-13." The pulmonary vessels expand with each inspiration, and contract during expiration, the result being an increased flow of blood from the right heart and the lungs: The dilated vessels, as Campbell puts it, " actually sucks the blood out of the right heart. The final factor, the splanchnic vasomotor mechanism, in preventing the gravitation of blood into the splanchnic veins, is an important one. Hill and Barnard have demonstrated that the splanchnic vasomotor mechanism suffices to combat this contingency, but when this mechanism is inhibited, as occurs when the splanchnic nerves are cut, a second mechanism is brought into prominence, viz.: Expiratory compressions of the abdomen occurring simultaneously with inspiratory thoracic suctions, the former squeezing, and the latter sucking the blood out of the splanchnic pool. The latter mechanism compensates, however ineffectually, in carrying out the circulation, and is referred to by Campbell as the " respiratory mechanism." That the latter mechanism is not as efficient as the vasomotor mechanism is evidenced by the fact that the effects of gravity may be entirely compensated for after the injection of curare, which paralyzes the muscles. Both mechanisms may be inhibited by division of the spinal cord at the first dorsal vertebra, and if the animal operated on be held with the head up all the blood accumulates in the splanchnic veins, and the empty heart ceases to beat; if, however, the abdomen of the animal is compressed, the blood is expressed into the heart, and the circulation is restored. With the foregoing facts at our command,

12

we are in a position to appreciate what I have called the *cardio-splanchnic phenomenon.*

If the lower sternal region, i. e., the part of the sternum contiguous to the heart, is first percussed in the standing and then again in the recumbent posture, one may note a decided alteration in the percussion tone; in the former attitude it is resonant or even hyperresonant, in the latter, it is dull or even flat. This is the cardio-splanchnic phenomenon. It may be elicited, but less pronouncedly when the patient is in bed and sits up. Vigorous compression of the abdomen will exaggerate the phenomenon in all instances. Not infrequently the deep or relative cardiac dulness will extend beyond the right border of the sternum. In no instance was this phenomenon absent, although hundreds of individuals were examined. It must be conceded that, in a few instances, the cardio-splanchnic phenomenon was only feebly expressed by mere attitudinal changes, yet re-enforcement of the maneuver by abdominal compression rendered its elicitation easy. A few forced inspirations will at once dispel the phenomenon, and it is likewise dispelled by the application of a vacuum cup to the abdomen. If the *liver* and *spleen* are percussed first in the erect and then in the recumbent posture, a decided variation in regional percussion is obtained. In the former attitude, the area of dulness is increased, in the latter, it is decreased, and the splanchnic area of dulness may completely disappear. These conditions are superadded to the cardio-splanchnic phenomenon. Primarily, it is necessary to adjust the discrepancy of my observations with those already accepted, and then to analyze the manifestations, which give genesis to the cardiosplanchnic phenomenon. Theoretically, one could at the outset assume that the situs of the heart, more nearly approaches the anterior chest wall in the erect than in the recumbent posture, indeed it is not only assumed but accepted by clinicians, that in the latter posture the heart falls away from the thoracic wall. Even Kingscote perpetrates a similar error by assuming that the preponderance of asthmatic seizures at night is caused by the recumbent posture, the dilated heart in this position causing it to impinge on the vagi. I have shown elsewhere the fallacy of this contention. By aid of the Röntgen rays, the triangular spaces in front and behind the heart are clearly defined, and the rays give undeniable demonstration of the fact that change of posture only slightly modifies, if at all, the area of these spaces; in fact, it may be observed in a number of instances, that when the patient assumes the recumbent posture, the anterior triangle is diminished and the posterior triangular space is increased in area, facts which contravene the contention that posture influences the relation of the heart to the chest wall. Again, percussional results are often influenced by the prejudicial preconceived ideas of the clinician. The skilled physician, in his interpretation of percussional phenomena, is guided not so much by the ear as by the *tactus eruditus;* thus palpatory percussion will yield results which would wholly escape the observer, who is influenced only by what he hears, and not by what he feels. In the elicitation of the cardio-splanchnic phenomenon, palpatory percussion must be our chief mentor. Others may contend that my lung reflexes (the lung reflex of contraction and the lung reflex of dilatation) and the heart reflex may account for the phenomenon in question, but all these reflexes have been carefully eliminated, and play no rôle in the cardio-splanchnic phenomenon. It is true that in the recumbent posture the areas of splenic and hepatic dulness become decreased, and this in accordance with the well known fact that change of posture influences the position of the lung borders, the so-called passive mobility of the lung borders. In the recumbent, the lower lung border descends about $\frac{1}{2}$ inch lower than in the erect posture. The decrease in the areas of hepatic and splenic dulness as associated signs of the cardio-splanchnic phenomenon takes into consideration only the deep or relative hepatic dulness, together with the additional fact, that the areas in question are diminished to an extent not to be accounted for by mere passive mobility of the lung borders. The cardio-splanchnic phenomenon is easy of explanation. In the erect posture, the blood leaves the right heart, which topographically is underneath the lower sternum, and tends to accumulate in the splanchnic area, whereas the recumbent posture opposes this influence of gravity. Pressure of the abdomen, which, in some instances must be vigorous, assists still further in expressing the blood from the splanchnic veins and sending it back to the heart. The same factors prevail with relation to the liver and the spleen, the amount of blood in the latter viscera being in direct proportion to the amount of blood contained in the splanchnic veins and in inverse proportion to the amount of blood contained in the heart. Forced inspirations hasten the output of blood from the heart, hence the almost immediate evanescence of the cardio-splanchnic phenomenon after vigorous breathing is executed. A word of caution is here necessary to those who seek the elicitation of the cardio-splanchnic phenomenon. If the latter is provoked, instruct the patient to conduct only superficial breathing and not to wholly suspend it, otherwise, the blood will accumulate in the right heart from this very maneuver. The exhaustion of air by means of a vacuum cup applied to the abdominal surface will decrease intra-abdominal tension, and will consequently increase the quantity of blood in the splanchnic veins, and in this manner the right chambers of the heart will become depleted. I have endeavored, by means of the Röntgen rays, to determine whether any of the maneuvers already suggested for provoking the cardio-splanchnic phenomenon in any way influence the diameters of the heart, and my investigations show that they do not. If the latter observation is correct, and there is every reason to believe that it is, how then can we account for the increased dulness of the lower sternum, the necessary concomitant of the cardio-splanchnic phenomenon. In the norm, the sternum contiguous to the site of the right ventricle of the heart, yields percussional resonance, which is caused in the main by the transmission of the percussion blow to the neighboring lung tissue. The percussion blow is propagated from $1\frac{1}{2}$ to $2\frac{1}{2}$ inches on the surface, and to a depth of about $2\frac{1}{2}$ inches. It is evident, then, that in the normal subject, the dulness of the right ventricle is not sufficiently pronounced to dampen the sound obtained from the vibration of air within the lung alveoli. It is, however, possible to conceive that if the right ventricle were sufficiently filled with blood, and this is capable of fulfilment without any increase in the dimensions of the chamber in question, that the normally resonant sound of the lower sternal region could become dull or even flat. Our final endeavor is to show the value of the cardio-splanchnic phenomenon in diagnosis and treatment. In estimating the size of the liver or spleen by percussion, we must pay due regard to the position of the patient, the amount of blood contained in the right heart and the vigor of respiration. The size of the liver is dependent in a measure on the amount of blood which it contains, and this has been estimated by Foster to be equivalent to one-fourth the amount of blood contained in the body. The skilled diagnostician will not find it a difficult task to demonstrate the reduction in the areas of hepatic and splenic dulness after repeated forced inspirations. Such reduction cannot wholly be accounted for by the opening up of atelectatic lung areas, for, in the case of the liver, percussional results should refer only to the deep or relative hepatic dulness. Supposing the object of our examination is an enlarged liver or spleen, and we wish to determine how much of this enlargement is due to passive or active hyperemia, and how much to hyperplasia of the connective tissues?

Percussion in different attitudes, repeated forced inspirations and abdominal compression will solve this question according to the methods previously advocated. If we wish to apply a crucial test, all that is necessary is to apply a vacuum cup to the abdomen, then in accordance with the fact already established, the liver and spleen would become enlarged. Supposing a patient presents himself complaining of pressure in the sternal region, the nature of such pressure if due to an enlarged right heart may be easily determined by application of the vacuum cup to the abdomen; the blood will be expressed from the heart to the abdomen, and the sensation of pressure will at once disappear. Let us further assume that we are confronted with an abdominal tumor and it is difficult to say whether such a growth is con-

nected with the liver or the spleen, the application of the
vacuum cup may solve the problem, for if the growth
in question is connected with the liver or spleen, the
latter viscera will show augmented dimensions, and con-
versely their areas will be diminished by vigorous compressions of the abdomen. If the differential diagnosis
rests between a pericardial exudate and a dilated heart,
the elicitation of the cardio-splanchnic phenomenon
would point to the existence of the latter condition.
Idiopathic syncope and the vertiginous attacks of Glenard's disease may be attributed to a defective splanchnic
vasomotor mechanism. Now, in the average normal subject the cardio-splanchnic phenomenon is fairly evident,
but in the conditions just cited, it is exaggerated. In
other words, the more perfect the mechanism, the less
pronounced is the phenomenon. There are a large number of respiratory affections which owe their dyspnea to
an overburdened right heart, and this is notably the
case in asthma. While I do not agree with Kingscote
" that a dilated heart is the essential cause of asthma,"
yet I do contend that an enlargement of that viscus is
operative in predisposing to an asthmatic paroxysm and
augmenting its severity. I have succeeded in arresting
asthmatic paroxysms, which failed to yield to the conventional methods by the application of a vacuum cup
to the abdomen. In these instances, suggestion probably
played no rôle, insomuch as the relief of the paroxysm
was coincident with the disappearance of the substernal
dulness. It is unnecessary to adopt the theory of Kingscote, that of a dilated heart striking the vagi, being responsible for the asthmatic attack, the overburdened
right ventricle being quite sufficient. Indeed, the pre-
dominance of attacks occurring at night, as well as the

dyspnea in cardio-respiratory affections, can be explained by the augmented blood supply to the right ventricle, as the result of the recumbent posture. In my opinion, the upright position intuitively assumed in orthopnea is not only due to the fact that the extraordinary muscles of respiration may work to better advantage, but also for the additional reason that the blood from the right heart is enabled to gravitate to the splanchnic veins.

Now in dyspnea from any cause, the implication of the heart in the production of this symptom may be gauged by expressing blood from the right heart by means of the vacuum cup to the abdomen. If the dyspnea is relieved, we have reasonable assurance that it is caused by an overburdened heart. Instances could be multiplied, showing how the cardio-splanchnic phenomenon may be employed in diagnosis, but the examples already cited will suffice. In treatment, the phenomenon suggests many possibilities in the direction of reestablishing the circulation and in relieving the heart when it is overtaxed. An accurate instrument for estimating the blood pressure is a trustworthy guide in determining the value of any physical maneuver, which has for its object cardiac stimulation. An equally efficacious guide is the cardio-splanchnic phenomenon, not only the phenomenon *per se,* but the degree of its demonstration. The precardial area of dulness is, as has already been intimated, not dependent so much on the approximation of the heart to the anterior chest wall, but rather to the amount of blood contained in the cardiac chambers. Inversion of the subject accentuates the cardio-splanchnic phenomenon and increases the dulness to the left of the lower sternal region, and diminishes it

over the latter area. In instances of syncope, it appears
to me, that the object achieved is not so much the determination of blood to the anemic brain as it is to the
determination of blood to the heart. I have sought to
devise some apparatus whereby continuous compression
of the abdomen may be effected in acute conditions de-
manding cardiac stimulation. The simplest means for
effecting this object is by means of a firm cushion applied to the abdomen and secured by a rubber bandage
or a broad strap, which permits of any degree of traction. Not infrequently continuous pressure, such as is
here described, gives rise to intereference with respiration, in which instance, one must content themselves
with paroxysmal abdominal compression.

The relief of an overtaxed right heart is suggested in
so many cardio-respiratory troubles that it may be apposite to select croupous pneumonia as a paradigm. There
are so many indications and contradictions cited by
writers for venesection in this affection that it is really
problematic whether bleeding is beneficial or harmful;
at any rate, its practice is purely empirical. It appears
to me that in the general management of the average
patient with pneumonia, the main object based on theoretic grounds, would be to preserve the quantity of
blood, for, after all, it is the chief stimulus for maintaining the cardio-pulmonary circulation and furnishes
the leucocytes, which are such important factors in conducing to a favorable issue. Instances do occur without doubt, where bleeding is a justifiable procedure,
but it would prove more effective if the patient could
be bled into his own vessels. The application of a
vacuum cup to the abdomen meets this emergency, and
should be employed, if only as a tentative measure,

should an overburdened right ventricle with its consecutive phenomena warrant its employment. If this maneuver is effective, it may be repeated, as it is a harmless and painless procedure.

NOTE 3.—BLOOD PRESSURE.

AFTER vigorous compression of the abdomen and coincident with the development of the cardio-splanchnic phenomenon, my investigations show, contrary to the observations of other clinicians, that the blood pressure falls. This is, in my mind, in accordance with two reasons: 1. By abdominal compression so much blood is suddenly expressed into the right heart that the latter finds great difficulty in discharging its contents; 2. Abdominal compression reflexly *inhibits the heart* action. Of the latter fact, I have convinced myself while executing the maneuver during the time the subjects were exposed to the X-rays. For this reason, in restoring cardiac action in syncope and other conditions, inversion of the patient or the application of a rubber bandage or leather belt around the abdomen, are safer procedures than abdominal compression. The question of blood-pressure in neurasthenia has received ample consideration from investigators, but nothing, however, of a practical value has been definitely elicited. The instruments for gauging blood pressure are erroneous, and so are the deductions even with an instrument of recognized accuracy. I regard the Riva Rocci instrument as more serviceable than the tonometer of Gärtner. The latter instrument is of little value on account of vasomotor changes in the finger of the patient, in hypertension and arterio-sclerosis. It is inapplicable in the negro. In hypertension and arterio-scerosis, clinical investigations have taught me aided by my *stethophonometer*, which enables me to accur-

ately gauge the intensity of the heart sounds that un-
reserved reliance placed on the tonometer as an instrument of precision in gauging blood pressure in arterio-
sclerosis is unwarranted by clinical evidence.

Arterio-sclerosis is by no means the general process
which is taught. On the contrary, it may be central,
peripheral or visceral. We may have a pronounced
type of intestinal sclerosis without evidence of its existence when gauged by the condition of the peripheral
arteries. I recall a case of arterio-sclerosis of the coro-
nary arteries of the heart which came to autopsy, the
arteries in question being as rigid as the stem of a clay
pipe, yet the individual during life showed no high
pulse tension, no cord-like, resistant, tortuous nor ribbed
radials; nor was there any evidence of heart hypertrophy
or accentuation of the second aortic sound.

It is usually taught that, when the tonometric figure
is low with clinical evidence of arterio-sclerosis, it is a
sign of failing heart power. The tonometer and other
like apparatus are constructed on the general principle
that, after the blood supply to a part is inhibited by
compression, the gradual removal of the latter will relieve the obstruction and, when the point is attained at
which the intra-arterial is greater than the extra-arterial,
or capillary, pressure, it is indicated by a gauge which
registers the blood pressure. Now, in arterio-sclerosis,
even the smallest blood-vessels (arteriocapillary fibro-
sis), are firm and unyielding, hence the compression
of such vessels for gauging blood pressure conduces to
erroneous results. I have frequently noted by the aid
of the tonometer an apparent increase of blood pressure,
notwithstanding the fact that cardiac auscultation nega-
tived the existence of the same. Three factors make up

the normal blood pressure, viz. : force of the ventricle, frictional resistance of the capillaries, and arterial elasticity. *If the heart is weak, as is manifested by an enfeebled second aortic tone, increased cardiac blood pressure cannot exist.* I am, therefore, constrained to conclude that in gauging blood pressure reliance should only be placed on cardiac auscultation.

It is generally conceded that of all the factors that make up blood pressure the resistance offered by the blood-vessels is one of the most important.

If the vessels are dilated, the pressure falls; if contracted, it will rise. The nervous mechanism which controls the blood-vessels is the vasomotor apparatus, and while the latter I concede may be reflexly influenced by irritation from the blood-vessels themselves or from the end organs of sensory nerves in general, we are inclined to forget that the vasomotor apparatus may operate independent of such influences. Emotions and the state of the mind in general, greatly influence the caliber of the blood-vessels through the vasomotor system of nerves. Take neurasthenics as a paradigm, and I have examined a large number of them at different periods under emotional influences, intense mental application, and when their brains were at rest and in each instance my results varied. Emotional influences and intellectual activity increased blood pressure, while mental inactivity reduced it. Again, increased cardiac pressure does not react equally on all the blood-vessels, and this, evidenced by the fact that the blood pressure in both radials is not always the same. Another factor influencing blood pressure is the *heart volume,* which is continually subject to reflex conditions (see Heart Reflex, appendix, note 8).

NOTE 4.—THE STOMACH AND COLON ON THE POSITION OF THE HEART.*

I HAVE referred elsewhere to the influence of a dilated stomach on the position of the heart. The accompanying illustrations show how easily the heart may be dislocated by artificial distension of the stomach. It is unnecessary

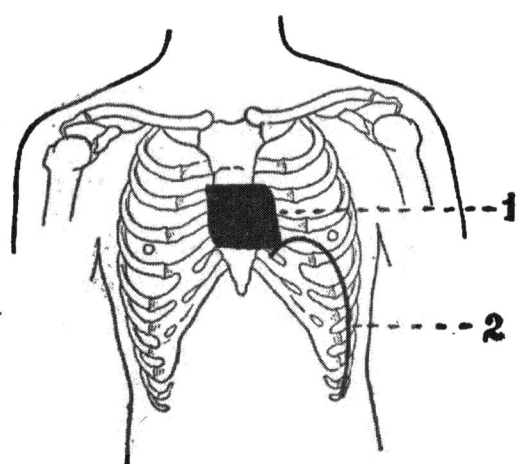

FIG. 13.—1, radioscopic appearance of the heart before administration of a Seidlitz powder ; 2, outline of the fundus of the stomach. The shadow of the heart area as shown in this and in fig. 14, is only correct in reference to the parts contiguous to the sternum as this bone obscures the heart silhouette.

to descant on the practical value of this observation. Heart dislocation from stomach dilation is associated with a circumscribed area of dulness in the left inter-

* *Medical Record*, Sept. 8, 1900.

scapular region. Over this area, bronchial respiration is heard. When the patient leans forward, dulness and bronchial breathing disappear, to reappear when the erect attitude is resumed. (Figs. 15, 17, 18.)

Leaning backward increases the area of dulness. The phenomena in question are produced by a dislocated heart compressing the lung, which fact is easily verified by the rays.

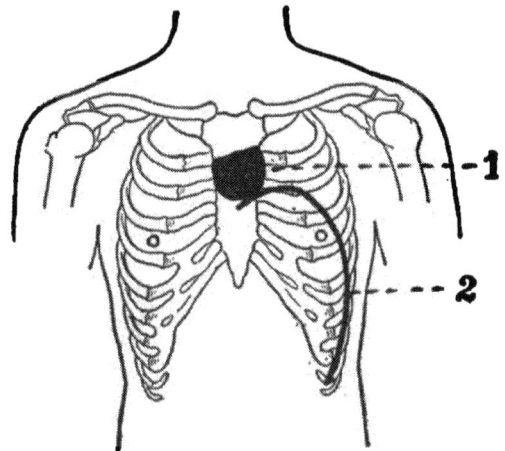

FIG. 14.—1, radioscopic appearance of the heart after administration of the Seidlitz powder ; 2, outline of the fundus of the stomach.

The foregoing syndrome may be reproduced synthetically by artificial distension of the stomach. An enormously distended heart may produce identical signs. Artificial insufflation of the colon is incapable of producing the same degree of cardiac luxation.

These observations explain the heart distress and pains after eating and from gas accumulations in neurasthenia.

NOTE 5.—PHYSICAL EXAMINATION OF THE LIVER.

THE conventional methods of examining the liver are by no means trustworthy. At the present time, palpation and percussion of the liver are the methods which will alone claim our attention.

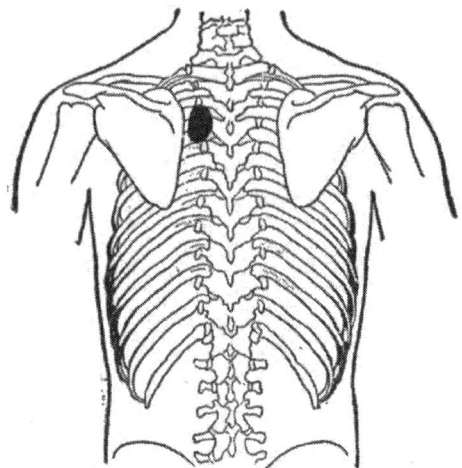

Fig. 15 —Patch of dulness in dislocation of the heart upward; patient in the erect position.

In palpating the liver, the physician proceeds exactly as if he were going to palpate his own liver. The patient should stand with body inclined very far forward, as shown in the illustration, then, with the fingers lightly bent, in a hook-like manner, they are insinuated

192

well under the curvature of the ribs ; it will be found
that, when the fingers are introduced under the ribs
in the right mammary line, they can be made to pene-
trate a considerable distance. The fingers being fixed,
in this situation and immobile, the patient is instructed
to take a deep breath and in accordance with the fact
that the liver alternately rises and falls during breathing, the border approaches the fingers during inspiration

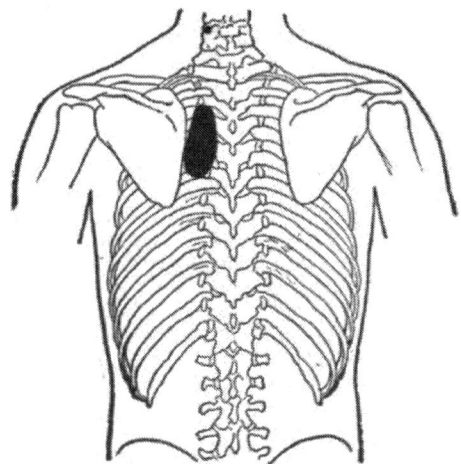

Fig, 17,—Patch of dulness in dislocation of the heart. Same patient leaning backward.

and recedes during expiration. This is my method of
palpation, and I have rarely known it to prove unsatisfactory. (See Frontispiece.)

In PERCUSSION OF THE LIVER, we have first to deal
with the topographic percussion of the upper and then
the lower border of the organ.

In PERCUSSION OF THE UPPER BORDER, I have already introduced to the profession a modified method of auscultatory percussion.

The modified method of auscultatory percussion, which I here advocate, is suggested after several years' experience in its employment. Its accuracy I have frequently controlled by skiascopy. It embodies the principle of transsonance. It is available in topographical

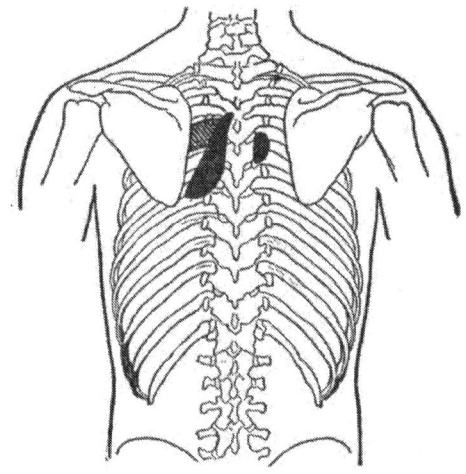

Fig. 18.—Fluoroscopic picture in dislocation of the heart. Black areas, shadows cast by normal heart. Shaded area, shadow of dislocated heart.

percussion, and for determining the density of the lungs after a method which will be presently described. Percussion transsonance is obtained when the thorax is percussed, either directly or indirectly, at a time contemporaneous with auscultation at some remote point. In my modified method of auscultatory percussion, the clavicles, sternum, ribs or vertebrae are percussed directly, i. e., without the interposition of the finger as a pleximeter. The percussion-blow is either light or strong, according to whether the superficial or deep dulness is to be elicited. If, for example, the area of cardiac dulness is to be obtained, the clavicle or manubrium sterni is percussed directly, and the stethoscope is gradually carried towards the organ in all directions from the lung. The area of the heart is at once indicated by a dull tone supplanting a resonant one. A similar procedure is carried out in eliciting the *upper liver-border*, and the splenic area of dulness. Lung-consolidation is also easy of elicitation by this method. If, for example, the trans-sonance of the apices is to be determined anteriorly, the stethoscope remains fixed first over one and then over the other apex, while immediate percussion is executed on a prominent vertebra. If the apices are to be auscultated posteriorly, the percussion-blow is limited to the manubrium sterni. It is possible by this method to outline the right auricle and the left ventricle on the posterior chest-surface, provided the patient is in the erect posture with body inclined slightly backward. The pectoral chest-piece of the stethoscope should possess a small caliber for the better object of demarcating the outline of organs. The fact must be emphasized that during the time this method of auscultatory percussion is executed the percussion-blow on some prominent bony structure must be continuous and uniform, while the stethoscope is carried toward the organ to be outlined. The percussion-hammer, recently designed by Dr. Heinrich Stern, of New York, will prove of great value in obtaining uniform results.

The drawbacks pertaining to my method are present only in corpulent individuals, in whom the well-padded, bony structures will not permit the percussion-blow to be conveyed to any distance. Another drawback, which is also present in the conventional auscultatory percussion is the inability to interpret the character of the percussion-sounds. This is, of course, a matter of practice. I cannot too highly extol this method, not only in topographical percussion, but also in determining the resonating qualities of the pulmonary tissue. I have elicited incipient lung-consolidation when the conventional methods have failed. I have also used this method for outlining the lower border of the stomach. The method of procedure in determining the latter, is briefly as follows: With the finger the lower ribs over the semilunar-shaped space of Traube are percussed, the stethoscope being fixed primarily in the hypochondrium in order to learn the character of the tympanitic tone. Then, while percussion is continued, the end of the stethoscope is gradually carried downward until the disappearance of the tone indicates that we have reached the lower border of the stomach.

PERCUSSION OF THE LOWER LIVER BORDER. The value of regional hepatic percussion needs no expatiation. No one, however skilled in percussion, can gainsay the insurmountable difficulties which beset the clinician in his attempts to demarcate an organ which is immersed in an atmosphere of tympanitic sound, and the edge of which does not exceed one centimeter in thickness. Take into consideration the facts that the contiguous viscera, stomach and intestines, vary in their degree of inflation and in the character of their contents, and we have additional factors which modify the accuracy of our percussional results. Posture and the phases of respiration are likewise disturbing elements. A liver may be very much enlarged, yet percussion as ordinarily practiced may give absolutely no evidence of

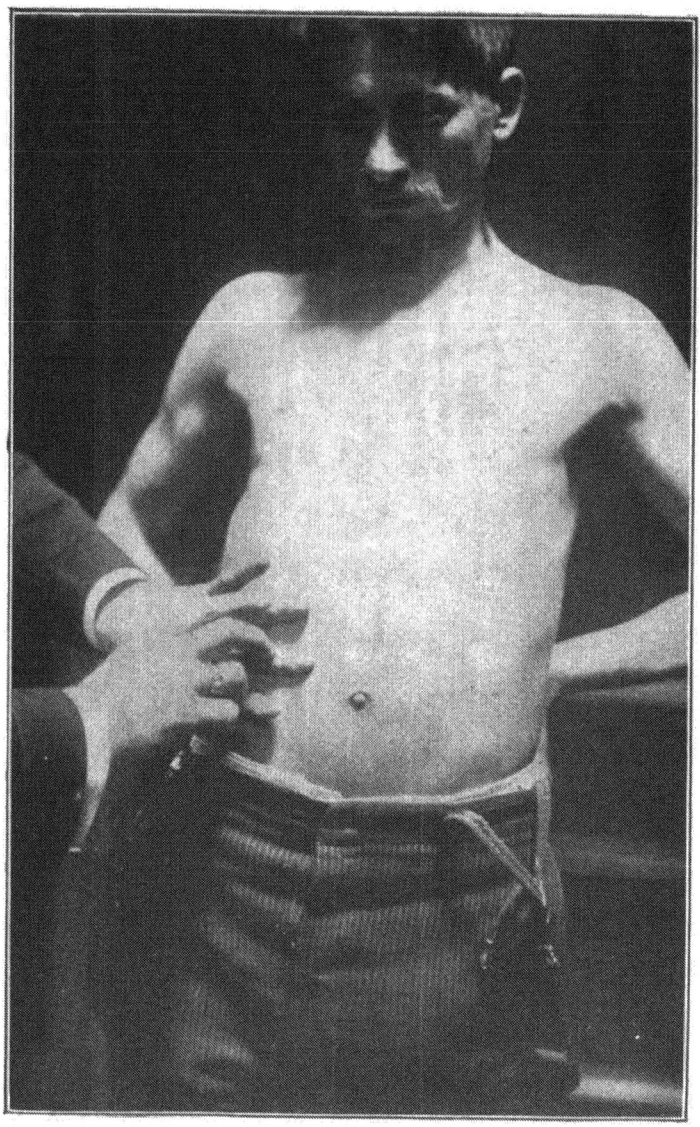

Fig. 19.—Author's method or percussing the lower liver border. The illustration does not show sufficient inclination of the body backward.

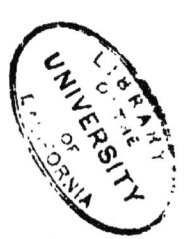

enlargement, if examination is made in the recumbent posture. A good rule to follow is never to declare the liver to be enlarged unless it is palpable ; but palpation may detect a liver which is dislocated, though not necessarily enlarged; and, again, rigidity of the abdominal parietes may negative the value of palpation.

In my " Manual of Diagnosis," I have referred to two methods of determining the lower border of the liver. One method is that described by C. Verstraelen, which is based on the fact that the intensity of the heart tones is well preserved over the entire hepatic region; at the lower border of the liver, however, the tones are suddenly lost; and in this way the lower liver border is determined. The abdominal walls must be relaxed, otherwise they will conduct the heart tones. This method I consider imperfect, as it is never of value if the cardiac tones are weak. Another method which I advocated in the same book is as follows: The patient is placed in a position favoring the approximation of the liver to the abdominal walls. This position is the knee-elbow o .e, or, if this is impossible, the erect posture, the body being inclined forward. The edge of a large coin is then deeply embedded in the abdominal walls, and the free edge of the coin is percussed lightly and shifted gradually upward from the tympanitic area until dulness is elicited. If this dulness represents the liver border, then, in accordance with the fact that the liver undergoes respiratory dislocation, the line of dulness will be lower during inspiration and higher during the act of expiration. The essential object embodied in this method is to verify the correctness of the percussion by dislocation of the organ during respiration. The latter method is relatively inaccurate, as I have had occasion to observe by controlling the percussional results by palpation in numerous instances where the latter method was easy of attainment.

A simple maneuver for mapping out the lower liver border on the surface of the abdomen is as follows: The patient is instructed to incline his body backward as far as possible, and, to relieve the tedium of the posture, the body is supported by means of the hands resting on the hips. If percussion, which must be light, is now attempted, the difficulty of determining the lower hepatic border is reduced to a minimum. (See Fig. 19).

If we analyze the rationale of this maneuver we will find that it involves a simple law in physics, viz.: that sound waves are best conducted by the medium in which they are produced. If the waves of sound are compelled to pass through media of different density, some of the waves will be lost by reflection, and the sound becomes correspondingly enfeebled. Solid bodies conduct sound better than air. If percussion of the lower liver border is executed in the conventional manner, the percussion sound first passes through the relatively-dense abdominal musculature and then through the air containing viscera before it reaches the liver. Theoretically at least, the percussion sound becomes enfeebled by the time it reaches the liver, inasmuch in the high pitch which reveals anything solid is dependent on the loudness of the percussion note, which in turn depends on the force exerted in percussion. We dare not employ a strong percussion sound in mapping out the lower hepatic border, for, by so doing, we set in vibration the air contained in the neighboring viscera and defeat the original object of our percussion, viz.: the elicitation of a dull sound. In the posture suggested, we approximate the surface of the liver to the abdominal parietes, thus affording a like medium for the transmission of the percussion sound. When patients are compelled to assume a recumbent posture the same object may be achieved by directing them forcibly to contract the abdominal muscles during the time percussion is executed. The results by the latter maneuver, however, are less accurate, though relatively better than by the conventional method of percussion.

Percussion of the liver while the abdominal muscles are contracted is a valuable means of ascertaining sensitiveness of the liver. It is a better method than palpation, which only admits of testing the sensitiveness of the lower border of the liver. I am cognizant of the dictum of Frerichs, who directed attention to the fact that contraction of the abdominal muscles will frequently yield a dulness on percussion, which is likely to be confounded with the dulness of the liver. This objection is, to my mind, purely theoretic. There is one condition, however, which demands consideration in percussion of the lower liver border and that is the presence of fecal concretions in the intestines contiguous to the liver border. The observation is undoubtedly correct that no one should rely on the results of liver percussion unless the bowels have been previously cleaned by free purgation. This teaching applies with all cogency to the entire abdomen. Experience has taught me the following simple method of determining the presence of fecal matter. If by palpation or percussion we suspect the existence of fecal stasis, massage of the suspected area for a few seconds will dissipate the dull percussion sound, which will then be supplanted by a tympanitic percussion tone. It is therefore imperative, before determining the lower border of the liver by the maneuver already suggested, to massage that region for several seconds.

There are two additional facts which deserve mention: First, the patient must be cautioned to take no inspiration before contracting the abdominal muscles, for by so doing the liver will be dislocated downward; second, in practicing percussion, the finger receiving the percussion blow must be firmly embedded in the abdominal wall; otherwise, the blow will not be directly transmitted to the liver.

After we have ascertained the lower liver border after the foregoing method, for corroborative purpose we may elicit the *liver reflex*. (See Appendix, Note 6.)

NOTE 6.—THE LIVER REFLEX.

MENTION has already been made in this work of various visceral reflexes to which I have first directed attention. All these reflexes are of great clinical importance, and in a therapeutic sense serve to explain the beneficial action of electro and hydrotherapy as well as other procedures applied to the skin for remedial purposes. The reflexes in question give objective demonstration how agents acting on the skin reflexly stimulate nutrition of the organs.

The *liver reflex*, which is here referred to for the first time, is elicited by irritating the skin contiguous to the lower liver border. The irritant may be a spray of ether, scratching the skin with the finger nail, or the blunt end of a pencil. Subsequent to any of these maneuvers, the lower liver border may be observed by percussion to recede a half-inch or more, depending on the degree of irritation. The sinusoidal current acts more efficiently in this regard than any irritant in causing the liver border to recede. This retraction of the lower liver border is dependent entirely on contractility of the liver itself, and not, as I have assured myself by repeated observations, by any influence on the amount of blood contained in the liver. I have already referred to the fact (see Appendix, Note 2), that the size of the liver can be graduated by the depth of respirations and compression of the abdominal wall.

The liver reflex is dependent on contraction of the muscular fibers contained in the fibrous coat of the liver which, as is known, invests the entire gland and at the transverse fissure, this coat turns into the substance of the liver with the branches of the portal vein.

NOTE 7.—THE CONDITIONS OF THE LUNGS ANTEDATING PULMONARY TUBERCULOSIS; BREATHING EXERCISES FOR DEVELOPING SUCH LUNGS.*

THE early recognition of pulmonary tuberculosis gives promise of its successful treatment, for, if there is one fact which the phthisiologist has demonstrated for curative medicine, it is the curability of phthisis. To-day the words of Brehmer are verified: *" Tuberculosis primis in stadiis semper curabilis."* The presence of shadows on the screen, as determined by the rays, is a sign equally as tardy as the recognition of tubercle bacilli in the sputa. We are here concerned only with skiascopic evidence, which betrays the disease at its very incipiency, even before physical signs are manifest. In this respect, the rays are of undoubted importance, and we possess . a means which permits of the very earliest possible diagnosis. Many of us, in our practice, meet with the phthisiophobiac, and we are now in the possession of means that will often rid that unfortunate individual of his fear. Of course, to depend on the rays alone for purposes of diagnosis would be to invite exclusivism, which would be fraught with danger to the catholic foundation on which diagnosis rests. There are two early signs to which I wish to direct attention, viz.: restriction of the excursions of the diaphragm, and the emphysematous X-ray appearance of the lungs. The physiologic diaphragmatic excursions vary according to whether the breathing is quiet or forced. In quiet

* *American Medicine*, March 1, 1902, and *Journal of the Amer. Mvd. Assoc.*

breathing, the extent of movement is about 1.8 cm. on the right, and 1.5 cm. on the left side; whereas, in forced breathing, the difference in the position of the diaphragm between forced inspiration and expiration, averages 6.7 cm. on the right and 7 cm. on the left side. Individuals with long thoraces show greater excursions of the midriff than deep-chested persons. The restricted diaphragmatic movements must be regarded as a very suspicious sign of phthisis, other things being equal. This sign, first referred to by Williams, of Boston, has received universal confirmation, but, to my knowledge, no theory has been advanced to explain its existence. I have sought elsewhere an explanation for this curious phenomenon, and I will briefly summarize my investigations, which gave birth to the theory that an emphysematous condition of the lungs exists in phthisis. Rokitansky noted that too voluminous lungs coupled with a small heart characterized the phthisical habitus. No one seemed to have contradicted this observation, and as a result it was soon relegated to oblivion. Brehmer revived and vigorously defended this hypothesis. The too voluminous lungs of Rokitansky and Brehmer are lungs which are practically the lungs of emphysema. In health, the percussion note of the lungs is resonant during inspiration and dull or even flat during expiration. In emphysema, the percussion note is unchanged during the two phases of respiration. This unchanged percussion note heretofore recognized in pulmonary vesicular emphysema is pathognomonic of lungs predisposed to tuberculosis, and in lungs already affected. Associated with the unchanged percussion sound there is an extension of the lung borders manifested by downward lung dislocation and diminution to the extent of obliteration of the cardiac and splenic areas of absolute dulness and diaphragmatic immobilization. As a rule, this lung emphysema in phthisis is limited to the lower lobes and is dependent on the fact that the air entering the respiratory tree travels in the direction of least resistance. Not infrequently, emphysema is associated with atelectatic zones. *If physicians were to depend on percussional dulness as an evidence of early phthisis, the affection would never be recognized; lung resonance, not dulness, is the early physical sign of phthisis.* The rays are invaluable in the recognition of the emphysematous condition. The lungs seem too large for the chest, the diaphragm is low and its excursions restricted. The lungs appear permanently bright, not alternately so as in their normal condition, and " statuesque " is about the best word to describe their appearance. It is interesting to observe parenthetically, how such lungs contribute to the development of phthisis. Defective pulmonary elasticity means some defect in the pulmonary elastic tissues. It may mean a congenital defect, as Cohnheim has observed, in a large number of cases of emphysema. A loss of pulmonary elasticity eliminates an important factor, not only in lung nutrition, but in the nutrition of the entire organism.

The exercises, then, in individuals with the phthisical lung, must be attempted not only in the direction of promoting inspiration, but what is even more important, in promoting the expiratory phase of respiration to expel the residual stagnant air in the lungs. The following simple method is serviceable: Two bottles, each capable of holding a gallon of water, are connected, as shown in the illustration.

The patient is directed, by expiration only, to transfer the water from one bottle to another. After a little

14

practice, with a single forced expiration, this is possible of achievement. I direct my patient to carry out this exercise, twice daily, each exercise lasting five minutes.

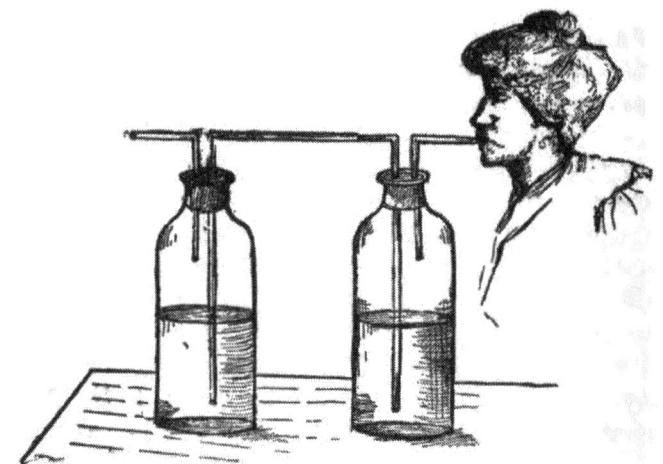

Fig. 20.—Arrangement of bottles for expiratory exercises.

The patient may also use with convenience and advantage a spirometer for exercising expiration.

This instrument will register the amount of air forced out of the lungs. The simplest and cheapest instrument for this purpose is the simplex spirometer.

NOTE 8.—THE HEART REFLEX.*

SOME years ago, I first directed attention to a phenomenon before undescribed, which I called the heart reflex. At that time I ascribed to it little clinical value, regarding it solely in the light of an interesting observation. Since then I have devoted considerable attention to this reflex, with the object of ascertaining its practical application. The result exceded my expectations. The heart reflex can be observed only with the Röntgen rays, the fluorescent screen approximating the anterior chest wall. The reflex is especially pronounced in children, and is best seen in adults· with thoraces scantily furnished with musculature and panniculus. If we irritate the skin in the precordial region by vigorous rubbing with a blunt instrument, a contraction of the myocardium is observed. The myocardial contraction is, as a rule,. more manifest in the left than in the right ventricle. The contraction thus induced is not sudden and of momentary duration, as I described in my original paper; on the contrary, its duration in children, on whom most of my observations were made, is not less, as a rule, than two minutes, and furthermore the myocardial recession continues even after the source of cutaneous irritation is removed. The degree of myocardial recession (heart reflex) varies greatly. In some persons it is scarcely perceptible, while in other individuals the heart may recede fully an inch on either side upon the first application of the cutaneous irritant. The accompanying illustration (Fig. 21) shows the degree of

* *Medical Record*, Jan. 5, 1901.

myocardial recession (line B) after cutaneous irritation; A representing the normal outline of the heart drawn on the fluoroscope.

This illustration is an exaggerated one, for, in the many examinations made by me, I have never been able to induce so marked a reflex. It is strange that in not a few instances the myocardial recession, although rarely

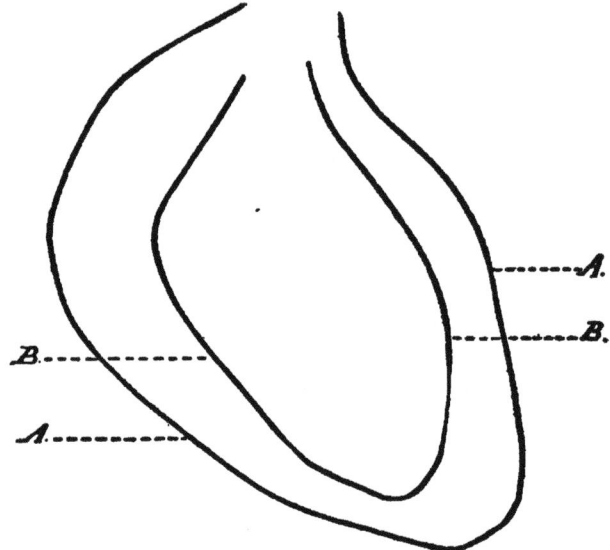

Fig. 21.—Heart reflex in a boy aged eight years. Duration of reflex, two and a half minutes.

absent when observed with a good X-ray apparatus, is but slightly marked. For this vagary, I am unable to account, occurring, as it does, in individuals with apparently healthy heart-muscle.

In Fig. 22 we note a rough reproduction from the fluoroscopic picture, demonstrating slight myocardial

recession confined solely to the left ventricle; A, representing the cardiac outline before and B after cutaneous
irritation; C is the upper hepatic line.

In my original paper, I advocated the rhigolene or
ether spray as the best cutaneous irritant; since then,
however, I have tested different modes of cutaneous irritation for clinical purposes, and I am now constrained
to conclude that friction of the skin by means of a rub-

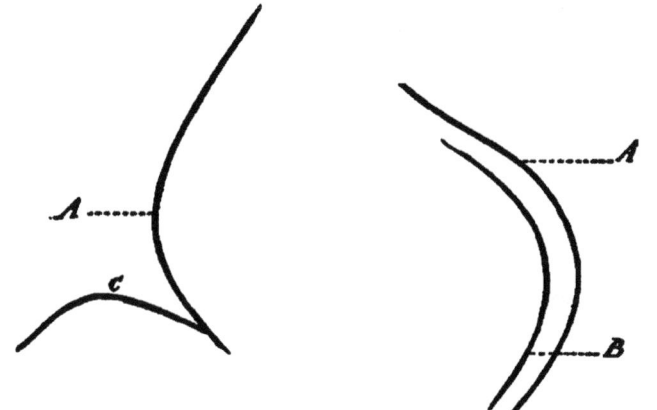

Fig. 22.—Heart reflex in a boy aged fourteen years. Duration of reflex,
fifty-five seconds.

ber (the ordinary pencil eraser is suitable) is the best
cutaneous irritant, for provoking this reflex.

The nearer we approximate the precordial region and
the more vigorous the cutaneous friction, other things
being equal, the more pronounced is the heart reflex.
The latter reflex may be slightly discharged, even
though the cutaneous irritant be applied to remote parts
of the body. In individuals with dilated hearts the
reflex is very evident, and of much longer duration than
in healthy hearts.

In a previous communication * I espoused the theory that the real factor involved in balneo and mechano-therapeutics (Schott) was dependent, not on the baths and exercises as such, but owing to the cutaneous irritation evoked by these maneuvers. In accordance with this theory I have, since this contribution, employed vigorous cutaneous friction by means of hand-rubbers obtainable at any drug store, after immersion of the patient in a warm bath for fifteen minutes; the warm bath augmenting the sensitiveness of the skin. By this simple and expeditious method, in chronic heart disease, I can adduce results emulating the conventional Schott method. Relief of dyspnea follows, there is reduction in cardiac volume, besides a marked reduction in pulse rate, with increase in volume and force.

The following conclusions may be formulated in reference to my method of treatment and that of Schott.

1. Lung dilation follows the exercise and bath treatment, the lung acting as an excretory channel for the overburdened heart.

2. The cause of lung dilatation is dependent on cutaneous irritation, induced by the exercises and baths.

3. A decrease in the volume of the heart also ensues, and is likewise provoked by cutaneous irritation.

In explanation of the heart and lung reflexes,† we all recognize the influence of the skin in physiological and pathological conditions. According to v. Preuschen, stimulation of the respiratory center is greater through the cutaneous nerves than through the vagus branches of the respiratory organs. In animals, which have been made apnœic, the application of cutaneous stimulation (cold water) induced stronger respiratory movements,

* *Medical News,* Jan. 7, 1899.   † Appendix, Notes 9 and 10.

and he concludes that mechanical cutaneous stimulation by flagellation, cold water, or the electric brush, is of the greatest value in stimulating the center of respiration.

The center for the inhibitory nerves of the heart is stimulated reflexly by centripetal nerves. In support of this physiological axiom we need only recall the "Klopf-Versuch" of Goltz, which demonstrates that striking the abdomen in animals will inhibit the heart's action.

I regard the heart reflex test as pathognomonic and far exceeding all other methods yet recommended in differentiating a dilatation of the heart from pericardial effusion. This is conceded to be one of the most difficult problems for the clinician. If, in a given case of increased cardiac dulness, which has been carefully outlined, we vigorously rub the skin of the precordial region by means of a rubber, and note after two minutes (the time necessary for the abolition of the lung reflex) a reduction in cardiac dulness, we are justified in concluding that we are dealing with cardiac dilatation and not with a pericardial effusion. Let me illustrate my meaning by reference to Figure (23). This is a rough reproduction of a reaction obtained in a young man with massive dilatation of both ventricles. A, represents the percussional area of the heart before cutaneous friction. The dark area represents the area of cardiac dulness after cutaneous irritation, and is caused not wholly by a reduction in cardiac volume, but also by the lung reflex of dilatation, which induces the lung to encroach on the area of cardiac dulness. After waiting two minutes, a time exceeding that necessary for the lung to recede, the percussional area B is obtained, which actually represents the decrease in the cardiac area (heart reflex). If pericardial effusion were present there would be some evidence of the lung reflex, but not of the heart reflex.

We have yet to learn the value of the heart reflex as an index to the condition of the myocardium.*

Since the publication of the foregoing I have studied†

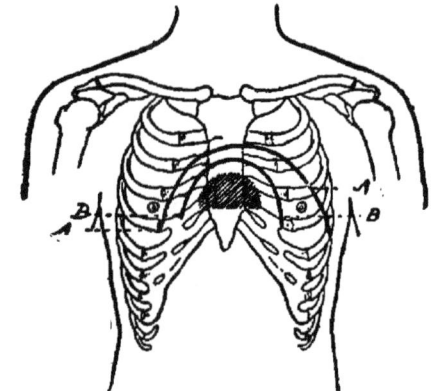

Fig. 28.—Illustration of heart reflex in Cardiac Dilatation. A, Percussional area of dilated heart. Dark area, percussional area after cutaneous friction. B, Percussional area, showing heart reflex persisting after abolition of the lung reflex.

the heart reflex as an index to the condition of the myocardium, and find in brief that when the cardiac muscle is beyond restitution in myocarditis and valvular diseases the reflex cannot be elicited. Heretofore this reflex was only observed in the transverse cardiac diameter, but it may also be noted in the sagittal diameter.

* The practical value of this reflex has been firmly established by the recent investigations of Merklen and Heitz in a paper before the " Société Medicale des Hospitaux " on " La Reflexe Cardiaque D'Abrams " (La Presse Medicale, Aug. 1, 1908.)

† American Medicine, Jan. 8, 1908.

The recognition of the heart reflex will often aid us in excluding the murmurs of a relative insufficiency. Here vigorous rubbing of the precordium will temporarily dispel the latter murmurs. One may elicit the heart reflex by irritation of more remote regions. I refer in particular to the nose. Some years ago, I directed attention to the pulmonary neurosis of dilation, which could be evoked in almost every healthy person by irritation of the nasal mucosa, and that such irritation was inoperative if the mucosa were previously cocainized. Later, I demonstrated that in persons suffering from asthma of presumable nasal origin, impacation of cotton in one or both nasal cavities would induce a typic asthmatic paroxysm. One may easily observe by aid of the X-rays that when ammonia is inhaled there is a decided recession of the cardiac ventricles (heart reflex), especially the left, and that this heart reflex may be more pronounced than when discharged through the skin of the precordium. Ether and chloroform produce a similar though less pronounced effect. With the nose closed, a similar though less pronounced effect of the vapors may be obtained, presumably by their action on the pharyngeal and laryngeal mucosa. In a few instances the vapors produced a veritable heart inhibition. I could observe no diminution in the intensity of the heart tones during the inhalation of the vapors, yet the accompanying sphygmogram (Figs. 24, 25) shows a decided difference in the output of blood into the general circulation before and after the inhalation of ammonia. These observations suggest the wise expedient of cocainizing the nasal mucosa before using an anesthetic, and further suggest the cogent necessity of anesthetizing the pharyngeal and laryngeal mucosa.

NOTE 9.—THE LUNG REFLEX OF DILATATION.*

ANOTHER interesting phenomenon is what I have denominated the "lung reflex." It illustrates the important fact that the respiratory area may be influenced indirectly by stimuli acting on the vagi. Elsewhere I have shown the value of the lung reflex in diagnosis. Here I will only consider its relation to lung development. In a contribution by Mocucci, the suggestion was made that when ether was sprayed over the left half of the abdomen, marked reduction in volume of the spleen was observed in 12 cases. In repeating the experi-

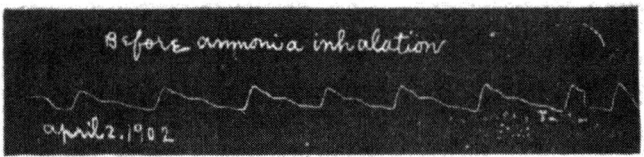

Fig. 24.—Sphygmogram, showing condition of pulse before inhaling ammonia.

ments, I likewise noticed a decided reduction in the area of splenic dulness in all individuals on whom this method was tried, irrespective of the fact whether enlargement of the spleen existed or not. Investigations convinced me that this diminution in the area of splenic dulness was not real, but only apparent. When the ether spray was directed over the region of the heart the percussional area of that organ was reduced at once; in fact, the superficial area of cardiac dulness could be obliterated by the maneuver. Similarly, when the spray was directed over the hepatic region the superficial area

* *American Medicine*, Feb. 15, 1902.

of dulness of that organ could be reduced at once. When the spray was directed over the border of the lungs posteriorly, the lung borders could be made to descend from two to four inches, dependent on certain conditions. It was further ascertained that dislocation of the lung borders by forced inspiration never approached the dilatation of the lungs produced by the

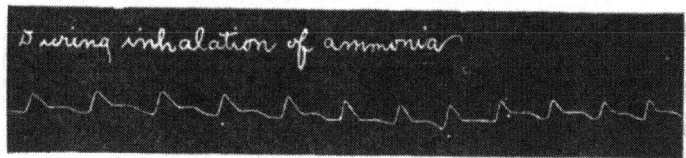

During inhalation of ammonia

Fig. 25,—Showing effects of ammonia during inhalation,

cutaneous application of the ether spray. Further experiments demonstrated in brief the fact, that the application of any cutaneous irritant, whether the latter be mechanic, chemic, or electric, would always induce acute dilatation of the lungs. Even in emphysematous individuals the application of a cutaneous irritant still further augmented the existing lung dilatation. The question naturally arose, by what means could we establish the fact that the application of any cutaneous irritant would cause acute dilatation of the lungs, a condition which, it may be mentioned parenthetically, is only of a few minutes duration. Such a hypothesis was made tenable by the aid of conventional physical signs, and the use of the fluoroscope. These aids show that when the skin is irritated by means of cold, by friction, or by a strong faradic current, lung dilatation will ensue. The degree of lung dilatation is dependent upon the character of the irritant, and the severity of its application. The response of the lung to dilatation is always greatest in that part of the lung contiguous to the source of cutaneous irritation. Lung dilatation may be recognized by the following physical signs: 1. Diminished respiratory excursions of the lung borders; 2. Extension of the pulmonary percussion note and obliteration of the cardiac and splenic areas of dulness; 3. Hyperresonance of the lungs; 4. Obliteration of the apex beat. Auscultation is of no value as a physical sign, inasmuch as the artificial dilatation does not last longer than three minutes after the source of cutaneous irritation has been removed. Lung dilatation spreads from the source of cutaneous irritation involving primarily circumscribed parts. In lungs, showing diminished resonance, the latter could always be increased by cutaneous irritation over the part percussed. The X-rays show how the brightness of the lungs is increased by cutaneous irritation. By gradually applying the irritant to different parts of the skin of the thorax, one may note that eventually the entire lung may be made to yield a more intense luminosity. This increased luminosity, however, does not last longer than three minutes in the average person, after which time the lungs resume their normal appearance.

In a number of measurements made during the study of the lung reflex after cutaneous irritation, I found the average dislocation of the lower border of the lung as follows:

Right sternal line............ .... 3¼ cm.
Right parasternal line.................... 3¼ cm.
Right mammilary line.................... 4 cm.
Right axillary line........................ 6 cm.

NOTE 10.—THE LUNG REFLEX OF CONTRACTION.*

I wish to direct attention to the Cherchevsky sign of early arteriosclerosis. This author contends that in normal conditions the diameter of the aorta varies at different times. It becomes dilated if the region over the arch is struck with the percussion hammer, while it shrinks in size if the blows are struck in the epigastrium. In arteriosclerosis it is impossible to produce these variations in diameter. The author has misinterpreted the phenomenon obtained by his maneuver. What he really elicits is a circumscribed lung contraction adjacent to the part struck on the chest by the hammer and the blow on the epigastrium merely causes the collapsed lung area to dilate, thus supplanting dulness by resonance. Dull areas may be obtained in other chest regions, especially in proximity to the sternum and spine, if vigorous percussion is conducted. For this purpose, I use a large wooden mallet and a pleximeter of felt. The circumscribed dulness thus induced lasts but a few seconds, but may be made to disappear at once by striking the epigastrium. Observed with the rays in a susceptible person, the phenomenon in question is a most interesting study. After the blow is struck, the adjacent lung area becomes gradually dark, showing that the air has been expelled from the lungs, whereas in a few seconds the lung area becomes bright again. This reflex cannot be obtained if the nasal mucosa has been previously cocainized, nor if the skin is irritated over

* *American Medicine*, Jan. 3, 1903.

the lung area, for then the counter reflex of lung dilatation is elicited. The phenomenon just described I have called the lung reflex of contraction to distinguish it from the lung reflex of dilatation.

The lung reflex of contraction has the same value in diagnosis and therapeutics as the counter reflex, but I will reserve its consideration for a future contribution. Suffice it to say at this time that we must hypothesize two distinct functions of the vagus, one which will enable it to dilate and fibers which can contract the

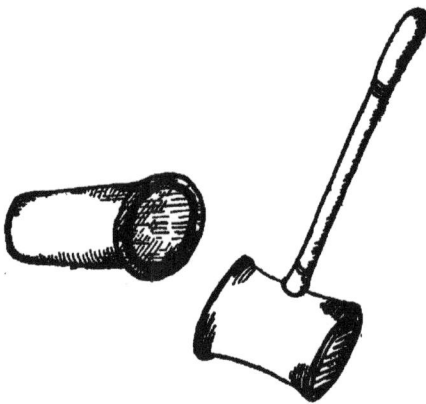

Fig. 26.—Mallet and pleximeter for eliciting the lung reflex of contraction.

bronchioles. This is the only hypothesis which permits us to explain the lung reflexes. Aufrecht has recently shown that the belief of only a circular layer constituting the musculature of the bronchi is wrong, and that by using the Biondi-Heidenhain stain a longitudinal muscular layer also exists. I contend, in view of this histologic fact, coupled with a knowledge of the lung reflexes and observations of asthmatics, that the theory of asthma must not alone be based on a spasm of the circular fibers of the bronchi, but on an inability of the weaker longitudinal fibers to expel residual air imprisoned by the circular fibers. In support of this theory I recall my observations with amyl nitrite. The primary effect of inhalation of this drug is to augment lung volume and then to diminish it so that its efficiency in arresting paroxysms of asthma is actually dependent

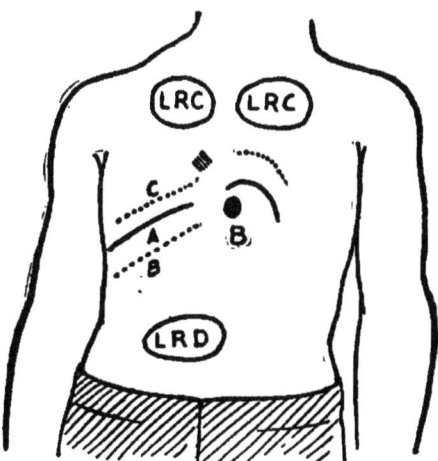

Fig. 27.—The lung reflexes of dilatation and contraction ; A, normal areas of heart and upper liver border respectively ; LRD, region for eliciting lung reflex of dilatation which, when struck, causes lung border to descend to B, and cover heart area almost to obliteration ; LRC, regions for eliciting lung reflex of contraction which causes lung borders to recede to C.

on contraction of the longitudinal no longer antagonized by the circular fibers. This action has its analog in the bladder musculature when, in consequence of a spasm of the sphincter vesicae, the weak detrusor vesicae cannot expel the urine, and ischuria spastica results.

Since the publication of the foregoing (*American Medicine*, Jan. 3, 1903, pages 11-15), I have been able to elicit the lung reflex of contraction after a manner which will bring both lungs simultaneously into a condition of contraction. My observations with reference to the latter maneuver I believe to be of great therapeutic value, and they are to be embodied in a work which is now in course of preparation.

NOTE 11.—SYMPATHETIC PAINS.

CLINICIANS have for a long time recognized the fact that in disease and irritation of the internal organs, superficial pain and tenderness are often referred to remote parts of the body. Thus in cardiac and aortic disease, pain is experienced between the shoulders; a carious tooth causes pain in the ear, etc. Head, who has thoroughly investigated this subject, shows that there is an intimate nervous connection between the viscera and definite skin areas, manifested by pain and tenderness appearing in sharply-localized regions on the surface when definite organs become disordered. He has also shown that in disease of the abdominal organs, pain and tenderness not only occur on the surface of the body, but the same pain and tenderness appear over certain areas of the scalp. He explains the topographic association of skin tenderness with visceral disease by assuming that the nerve-supplies of the parts so related find their origin within the same segment of the spinal cord: Thus, when a painful stimulus is applied to a part of low sensibility like an abdominal organ, which is in close central connection with a part of much greater sensibility, the pain produced is experienced in the part of higher sensibility rather than in the part of lower sensibility to which the stimulus was actually applied.

Two factors are recognized by biologists as responsible for the actions and character of the living organism, viz.: *heredity* and *environment*. It is often difficult to determine whether a specific vital phenomenon is a result of inheritance or a reaction to environmental influences. Resemblance to ancestors is an acknowledged product of inheritance.

Galton has estimated that, of the total heritage of the child, each of two parents contributes one-fourth, each of the four grandparents one-sixteenth and the remaining one-fourth is handed down by more remote ancestors. The congenital resemblances may be *anatomic*, as expressed by physical resemblances, (facial features, stature, color of hair and eyes) or by anatomic defects of the eyes, cleft palate, monstrosities, etc. They may be *physiologic*, as expressed by characteristic gestures, peculiarities in gait, tendency to obesity, to longevity, and to certain diseases, such as gout, asthma and epilepsy. They may be *psychologic*, as expressed by artistic and moral qualities, traits of character, temperament, mental diseases and proclivity to crime and suicide. Characters transmitted from grandparent to child and never appearing in the parent are referred to as *latent characters*. Latent characters are very often associated with sex. Character latent in the intermediate ancestor is evidenced by the appearance of the female characteristics in castrated males, and of male characteristics in females with diseased ovaries. Latency is further expressed by *atavism* or *reversion*, terms which refer to the appear-

226

ance in an individual of peculiarities known only in remote ancestors, but not in the parent of the individual.
Darwin instances many examples of reversion, such as
the frequent appearance of stripes upon the legs of
the mule, the latter being a hybrid from the horse
and the ass, both of which are comparatively unstriped,
but are unquestionably descended from a striped zebra-
like ancestor. The same writer attributes the degraded
state of half-castes to reversion to a primitive savage
condition, which, usually latent in both civilized and
savage races, is made manifest in the offspring that results from the union of both. *Regeneration* is likewise
a phenomenon of heredity, and refers to the capacity of
the organism to replace parts lost by accident or destroyed by disease. The regenerative power becomes
progressively stronger as we descend in the scale of animal life. Thus a newt may replace a lost leg, a crab
a lost claw, the snail, an eye stalk or eye. A hydra may
be cut into pieces and each piece may re-grow into a
complete hydra. If an earth-worm is divided, one-half
may regenerate a new half which is in every respect
complete. The *Inheritance of disease* is not always the
transmission of an actual parental disease; on the contrary, a diseased parent may produce offspring that are
constitutionally weak, and the disease of the parent may
later on attack the constitutionally weak body. Without entering into a discussion of the theories of inheritance, modern biologists attribute much truth to the
theories of *preformation* and *epigenesis.* The first is
practically the Darwinian theory of *pangenesis.* It assumes that the cells or units of the body increase by
cell-division or proliferation, retaining the same nature,
and that they ultimately become converted into the

various tissues and substances of the body. Aside from this means of increase, the cells throw off minute granules which are dispersed throughout the whole system; that these, when supplied with proper nutriment multiply by self-division and are ultimately developed into units like those from which they were originally derived. These granules are collected from all parts of the system to contribute the sexual elements, and their development in the next generation forms a new being; but they are likewise capable of transmission in a dormant state to future generations, and may then be developed. Their development depends on their union with other partially developed or nascent cells which precede them in the regular course of growth. The granules are thrown off by every unit, not only during the adult state, but during each stage of development of every organism. The granules in their dormant state have a mutual affinity for each other, leading to their aggregation into buds or into the sexual elements. Therefore, it is not the reproductive organs or buds which generate new organisms, but the units of which each individual is composed. Thus the theory of Darwin explains the regeneration of lost parts by supposing that the granules of the part in question are disseminated throughout the body and have only to unite with the nascent cells at the point of new growth. The theory also explains reversion by supposing that the granules lie dormant in one generation and develop in the next. It further explains how acquired variations may be cogenital, since an altered part throws off altered granules and by collection of these in the germ sells the alteration may be transmitted, thus explaining the transmission of acquired characters. The theory of Epigenesis assumes that there is no preformation in the germ cells, but rather a lack of organization which during growth, under guidance of a mysterious power, gives place to differentiation and the appearance of definite parts. Much experimental work is now being done, chiefly on marine invertebrates, to determine how many of the characteristics of the offspring are due to the original qualities of the germ plasm and how much to the physical, chemical and physiologic phenomena of the immediate environment of the developing embryo. Applying the foregoing facts to the heredity of nervous diseases, we have, first of all, the fact, that a nervous disease is rarely directly inherited. What is really transmitted is a general predisposition to nerve disease, the subjects having inherited unstable and irritable nervous systems, they possess, in other words, what is known as a *neuropathic constitution*. Individuals of genius are neurotics, as a rule, and may beget a progeny with neuropathic constitutions, but such a tendency would be less likely, if one of the parents were of a phlegmatic temperament. Shock or injuries to the mother during the early months of pregnancy may lead to nervousness in the offspring. There are so-called *family diseases* which may be transmitted by direct inheritance from parent to child, or may skip a generation. In the latter instance, we have a manifestation of atavism which rarely goes back more than two generations.

Morbid traits, peculiar to a family, may reappear at the same age in the offspring, but if such traits show a tendency to disappear with each successive generation, they appear later in life in the descendants. If such traits become exaggerated, they appear at an earlier age in the descendants.

NOTE 18.—THE SINUSOIDAL CURRENT.

THE use of the Sinusoidal current in Electro Therapeutics is of comparatively recent introduction, and even now its effects are not fully appreciated by physicians.

The character of this current, when produced with proper apparatus, approximates a true alternating current curve.

The use of this apparatus is to produce anaesthetic effects on the Sensory and Motor nerves; and by it, stimulation to muscular action can be obtained without the accompanying pain to the patient, which is attendant on the uses of other currents, if used in the same proportion. In consequence, a greater quantity of electricity can be used than with the induction coil, so that more physiological action of the muscles is obtained than by other methods. Further, the more nearly the curve of the current approaches to the true sinusoidal, the less will be the effects resulting from polar action, thereby avoiding electrolysis and cataphoresis.

The current is also found to be useful as a means of improving the nutrition of muscular tissue, and also for general muscular weakness. It also has the peculiar property of allaying pain, if the alternations are sufficiently rapid.

There are four forms of this apparatus in use by physicians. The first form is obtained by taking the current direct from alternating lighting mains, moderating the strength by controlling apparatus. The number of alternations per minute are limited to that of the central station.

The second form is obtained by cutting the wires of any direct current motors, and obtaining one complete alternation for each revolution. The disadvantage of this apparatus is that the number of alternations is limited to the speed at which the motor can be operated, usually not exceeding 4000 to 6000 alternations per minute, and has the further disadvantage that the lines of magnetic force are cut by the revolving coils unequally so as to form an irregular curve, and in many cases the apparatus is so designed that a change in the speed varies the strength of the field.

The third form is obtained by using a direct current motor to run a magneto-electric machine, the alternations of which are limited to the speed of the motor operating the magneto, unless belting is used, then the inequalities of the belt produce serious inequalities in the current.

The fourth form has been invented by Dr. Kennelly, associated with Mr. Thomas A. Edison, and is designed to secure a true sine curve, a constant field, and increase the alternations sufficiently to obtain anaesthetic effects; and constructed so that when belted to the motor it will obtain a frequency up to 150,000 alternations per minute. But this introduced belting causes irregularities which to overcome the owner of the Kennelly patents has improved by designing and having built a motor that will develop an equally high frequency, using a direct connected couple; thus eliminating all belting troubles.

The magnetic field of the Kennelly apparatus remains

constant at all speeds, but may be varied in strength as desired.

The strength of current in patients' circuit is controlled by a high resistance rheostat.

BIBLIOGRAPHY.

1. *Shattuck Lecture*—"Not the disease only, but also the man."
2. *Journal American Med. Assoc.*, March 7, 1903.
3. *Medical Record*, Nov. 22, 1902.
4. *Journal of Morphology*, Boston, 1892.
5. *Clinical Lectures on Neurasthenia*, 1902.
6. *Sexual Neurasthenia*, Beard and Rockwell, 1895. New Ed. 1902.
7. *Weiner Klin. Wochenschrift*, Nos. 2, 4, 5, and 7, 1898.
8. *Corresp. f. Schweizer Aerzte*, No. 6, 1897.
9. *Medical Record*, Feb. 5, 1898.
10. *Medical News*, June 25, 1898.
11. *The Lancet*, Jan. 21, 1903.
12. *Auto-intoxication in disease*, 1894.
13. *Ueber habituelle Stuhlverstopfung deren Ursache u. Behandlung*. Berlin, 1891.
14. *Blutdruck und Darmatonie*, 1894.
15. *Clinical Lectures on Neurasthenia*, 1902.
16. *Croonian Lectures : British Medical Journal*, vol. 1895, p. 6.
17. *Archives Gén. de Méd.*, Dec. 1892.
18. *Wiener Klin. Wochenschrift*, June 16, 1898.
19. *American Medicine*, Feb. 15, 1902.
20. *Text-book of Nervous Diseases*, 1901.
21. *Clinical Lectures on Neurasthenia*, 1902.
22. *Deutsch. Med. Wochenshrift*, 1896, pp. 53, 78, 87.
23. *Revue des Maladies de la Nutrition*, 1896, pp. 723, 724.
24. *Journal of Physiology*, vol. xxi, p. 323.
25. *Respiratory Exercises*, 1898, p. 12.
26. *Journal of Physiology*, vol. vii, p. 202.
27. *Lancet*, 1894, vol. i, p. 587.
28. *Respiratory Exercises*, p. 86.
29. *Phil. Med. Journal*, Dec. 7, 1901.
30. *Volkmann's Sammlungen*, Nos. 115, 116, 1895.
31. *Archiv. f. Verdauungsk*, Bd. ii, 1896, pp. 285–295.
32. *Text-book of Physiology*, 1898, p. 71.
33. *Therapeutic Gazette*, July 15, 1901.
34. *Halliburton's Kirke's Physiology*, p. 537.
35. *Verhandl. d. Congr. f. innere Med.* 1897, pp. 521–523.
36. *Journal of Physiology*, vol. xxi, p. 323,

INDEX.

Lightning Source UK Ltd.
Milton Keynes UK
UKHW021232200521
384060UK00004B/832

9 781376 374681